SARAH KEY

BACK IN ACTION

SARAH KEY

BACK IN ACTION

Do you have backache?
This book will put it right

CENTURY
London Sydney Auckland Johannesburg

This edition published in 1991 by Century
An imprint of Random Century Group Ltd
20 Vauxhall Bridge Road, London SW1V 2SA

Random Century Group Australia (Pty) Ltd
20 Alfred Street, Milsons Point,
Sydney, NSW 2061, Australia

Random Century New Zealand Ltd,
9-11 Rothwell Avenue, Albany,
Auckland 10, New Zealand

Random Century Group South Africa (Pty) Ltd,
PO Box 337, Bergvlei 2012, South Africa

The right of Sarah Key to be identified as the author of
this work has been asserted by her in accordance with
the Copyright, Designs and Patents Act, 1988.

British Library Cataloguing in Publication Data
Key, Sarah
    Back in action .-Rev. ed.
    1. Man. Back. Backache. Relief. Alternative methods
    I. Title
    616.7306

    ISBN 0-71 26-4990-5

Printed and bound in Great Britain by
Butler & Tanner Ltd, Frome and London

To my four children;
Jemima, Harry, Freddie
and Scarlett

ACKNOWLEDGEMENTS

When the first edition of *Back in Action* was finally completed and in the bookshops, I began to lament my lack of acknowledgement of the people past and present who helped me turn my youthful fascination with backs into a consuming interest, indeed a whole way of life. With that in mind, and the opportunity offered by this new edition, I would like to express my thanks to some special individuals.

There were some who, it could be said, gave this young hitch-hiker lifts along the way: Alec Sinclair, the New Zealand doctor at King's College Hospital in London, who taught me the first essentials of spinal manipulation; Greg Grieve who, with his mellifluous delivery, brought language and lyricism to the dry old world of orthopaedic medicine; Geoff Maitland, the Australian pioneer and 'Prophet... save in his own land', who put manual therapy on the map; and finally, Lance Twomey and Nikolai Bogduk, the brilliant Australian academics who have brought critical analysis to the fore, helping background an art with science but not necessarily turning it into one. And then there are the patients — not just bodies but real men and women who placed their faith and trust in me. They are the ones who really taught me.

Sydney, February 1990

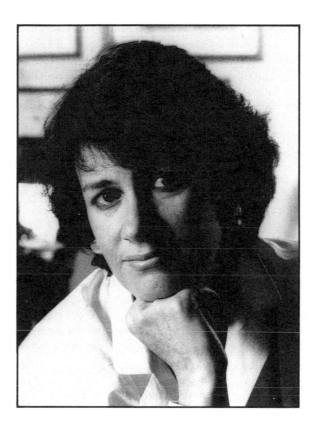

Sarah Key was born and brought up in Australia. She came to London as a young back-packer in 1973. In 1976, as a result of her consuming interest in the human spine, she opened her own physiotherapy centre in the Harley Street area of London.

She now treats backs on both sides of the world, spending a lot of her time in Sydney, but she returns to the UK throughout the year to tend to patients here.

Sarah Key is married to a Sydney lawyer and has three small children.

Contents

FOREWORD

British industry is said to lose more man-hours of otherwise productive time through 'bad backs' than through any other cause, yet I am told that the understanding of human back disorders has hardly advanced at all in the last 30 years. So it is encouraging to encounter the refreshingly direct approach which Sarah Key, as a physiotherapist, adopts in this interesting and challenging book. Speaking directly to the sufferers, and there must be literally millions of us who do suffer from time to time in this way, she explains the problems using easy-to-understand layman's terms.

Of course, there will always be people who disapprove when collective conventional thinking is challenged, in the field of medicine or any other area for that matter, but there must surely be a place for common sense and a 'natural' non-invasive approach, based on an intimate knowledge of the musculo-skeletal system, alongside the more conventional treatments. This book certainly suggests that there is, as do many people who have been helped by the techniques of manipulation which it advocates. At this point I must stress that I am writing as someone whose back has been infinitely improved by Sarah Key's ministrations, not to mention my arm ...! However, the treatment also involves a great deal of hard work and application on the part of the patient!

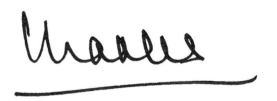

INTRODUCTION:

I wanted to call this book 'About Backpain without the Bullshit' but they wouldn't let me.

HOW THIS BOOK CAME ABOUT

In March 1973 I left my native Sydney to go 'overseas'. There is nothing unusual about that; lots of young Australians do it. At the airport I cried buckets of tears, but I knew I had to go. I had something to do and I knew I had to leave to do it. Sometimes you have to leave to set free a murmur inside. That very murmur might instantly be swept away, lost in a chilling eddy of thin foreign air, but at least it had a chance away from the close scrutiny of 'home'. It is easier to make a go of things on someone else's pitch. I was going to London.

I made my journey to England overland across Africa. We were travelling in long-wheelbase Land Rovers and making a very slow job of it. We were inching across the northern part of Zaire when one evening as the heat was fading from the day, I sat idly watching as one of our party fell asleep upright in her seat. Her head hung heavily to one side as the vehicle lurched clumsily over red earth roads which were narrow and deeply pot-holed and overhung with a dense tangle of jungle greenery. We camped that evening, and the night passed, but the next morning she woke barely able to move her neck. Because I was a physiotherapist, the group looked to me to 'do something' and, frankly, I could do nothing. Beyond offering some vague form of massage and a few words of solace, I was as much help as anyone else in the group. I felt useless. Like so many people who spend their life grappling with a spinal problem, I, too, was in the dark, wandering in a wilderness, completely at a loss to know what to do for the best.

But a clear distillate of purpose pooled in my mind. I realised then with absolute clarity what I must do. In that stiff spine something stiffened within me — the resolve quietly to pursue a single goal. I was not ambitious; I just never changed my mind. My mission was to find out a thing or two about the human spine, those delicately poised mechanisms that so often go wrong. Why? And were there not some effective simple measures to help one that had gone wrong? Or would there always be only two options: either do nothing or contemplate drastic measures? Surely there must be a wide welcoming middle road somewhere for the finding.

Looking back I often think that my personal road to Damascus was in the thick of the jungle, deep in the heart of Africa. The longer we dallied there, the keener became my enthusiasm.

I flew into London from Tunis to be greeted by the 1973 heatwave. It was quite unlike the London I came to know. Everyone was busying about with great cheeriness and expectation, as people do in the Northern Hemisphere with the smile of unaccustomed sun on their backs.

It was the end of July and it was hot. In the Tube during the rush hour it was every bit as uncomfortable as it had been in the Central African Republic two months earlier. But I remember being exhilarated with the new-found purpose I had discovered in life. This exciting city, with red double-decker buses and legendary place-names like Pall Mall and Park Lane, was to be my home for many years. It was to be the maze I would wander through in my search for knowledge.

I was as poor as a church mouse. I lived with an unusual collection of itinerant Australians in a cold and echoing house in Kilburn, north London. We were a mixed bag of people. One was a barmaid, another was a builder's labourer, another was a reporter/photographer for the *Australian* newspaper in London, others were working in Harrods selling stockings. Just about all of them earned a better salary than I did. It was pretty hard to earn less than thirty pounds a week. Physiotherapy was a poorly rated trade.

As winter drew in around us, we could barely afford to have the single gas-fire burning in the living room. The kitchen was so cold in mid-winter that we had to don overcoats and mittens if we were planning on an extended session. Any friend or acquaintance who dossed down on the floor and did not make his contribution to the gas bill was instantly an outcast.

I went for various job interviews; there were many hospitals crying out for staff, but I only wanted to go where I could glean some knowledge. I had heard that the Royal National Orthopaedic Hospital in Great Portland Street was the place to be, but there were no vacancies there at the time and I did not get to work there until two years later in 1975.

Meanwhile I fell sick with infectious hepatitis, a legacy of my trip through Africa. For three weeks I was barricaded into a single room in the Middlesex Hospital in Mortimer Street and barrier-nursed. My only company during that time was a book I had asked someone to buy for me. It was *Vertebral Manipulation* by G. D. Maitland, and I read it from cover to cover throughout that lonely time.

That book supercharged me with adrenalin. I just could not wait to get out there. I was dying to be let loose amongst that population suffering from painful backs. According to this book, it all seemed so logical, not at all the vexing mystery so many felt it to be. As a result, I didn't care where I worked, just as long as it was in an outpatient department where patients obligingly presented themselves with their problem spines for me to work on.

My first job was at the St Leonard's Hospital in the East End of London. It was probably one of the most run-down and neglected hospitals in the country. I remember that one would walk straight from the front reception hall of the hospital into a vast staff dining room with walls lined to the ceiling with pale blue tiles so that the place resembled a huge fish-tank. A few sleepy hospital porters sat reading newspapers and muttering to one another in a monotone, and nobody could direct me to the physiotherapy department. However, I was as happy as a sandboy to be working there. Long-suffering patients who had previously either been turned away with a sad shake of the head, or, worse still, had been treated with heat and exercises without relief, doggedly re-presented themselves to the doctors in the outpatient clinics in the hope that modern medicine had finally conjured up some form of relief, even if that form was me, tentatively feeling my way around in backs with the book open at the right page.

In 1976 I opened the doors of my own private consulting-rooms in Weymouth Street, in the Harley Street area of London. They were two rooms on the second floor with a clanky old lift with a concertina wire-grille door. The rooms themselves were completely bare but pleasant and airy. The contents were one desk, two chairs and a treatment couch. This and a pair of hands — the simple tools of the trade. The way seemed clear ahead. I had nothing to lose. I still had no money. I calculated that I only had to see a few patients per day to be able to pay the rent and still have a bit to live on, so things could only get better. Besides, it was a far better arrangement for me to see the increasing numbers of patients being referred by the consultants from the National Orthopaedic Hospital at a proper professional place, rather than at their homes or in hotel rooms.

And the English are a very easygoing bunch; they are pretty good to the Aussies. They smile on us in mild amusement, rather like an indulgent benefactor observing an unruly child. A decade and a half later my clinic is bigger. The voices of the workforce have the unmistakably level tone of the Australian drawl. The walls are no longer bare. They are cluttered with photographs of New South Wales, whether it be Sydney Harbour as Clive James describes it — water sparkling in the sun like crushed diamonds under skies the texture of powdered sapphires — or the smoky blue hills of the Hunter Valley, or the black silence of Pittwater at dawn. I have homes in both London and Sydney and I spend many hours in the air, travelling back and forth between the two.

I have learnt that there is no shortage of back suffering. I have also learnt that lots of back problems can be rectified by tinkering around with the spinal joints with the hands. Yes, the hands — that most ancient form of healing, so long relegated to a therapeutic backwater. I have learnt that there is some hope for the back sufferer who was sent away with a bottle of pills or idly despatched to the physiotherapy department for heat treatment or massage in the feeble hope that this would loosen things up a bit, only to find that once the heat and enthusiasm had died down the pain was there just as persistent as ever.

In April 1984 I wrote the first draft of this book. I did it because I know that everyone who has a back problem has questions to be answered. Furthermore, many of those questions are common to every sufferer and all of you have a hard job getting any satisfactory answers. In short, the back sufferer gets a pretty rough deal from the medical profession.

I know that anyone who has backpain talks about it all the time. There is a huge league of fellow-sufferers out there who share a kind of camaraderie about their mutual problem. The grapevine is enormous, and lots of information and even more misinformation is swapped incessantly. Back specialists talk in elite medical language, and patients misquote the specialists. Out there in the world there is a veritable sea of inaccuracies about backpain — the worst being that it is incurable. This book is based quite simply on the premise that a bit more information would help the cure. Questions need to be answered, because an illness diagnosed is half-cured. Surely it is not for you to have the problem and for we specialists to do the worrying about it!

But my greatest misgiving about writing this book is the anticipated furore from the close learned circle who may well be offended at an irreverent approach to unveiling the mystery. But to date, for fear of being wrong, nobody says anything! Furthermore, the precious little knowledge that we do have is too jealously hoarded by the guardians of the speciality. Too long has it been the case that unless we spoke in barely intelligible quasi-scientific medical jargon about a problem we could not be relied upon to know what we were talking about.

You will find that bits of the text are fairly technical. You have no option but to plough on through that; it is simply not possible to discuss a structure as complicated as the spine in a series of monosyllables and pretty pictures.

Knowing all that, here I go, grasping the nettle and biting the bullet . . .

1

WHY IS BACKPAIN SO COMMON?

Backpain certainly is common, but the truth of the matter is that backs are only painful if they are failing to work properly. Pain exists for a reason. If all the joints of the spine run smoothly, there is no pain.

If you wonder why it is so important that the back lets us know so quickly that things are not right, the answer is simple. It is because the longer that spinal function faults go unchecked, the more widespread the strain suffered by the skeleton as a whole. It does not do us any good at all to try to operate as a purposeful working system if the fundamental background activity of the system is below par. The role of pain is to bring the faulty function to the forefront of our consciousness to enhance the chances of the fault being fixed.

An active well-working spine provides effortless gross and fine adjustments in the stance of the frame so that the stage is set for all deliberate fruitful activity. If there is a fault in this background function, we are put at a physical disadvantage and *all* our skills become handicapped. Although we may not be conscious of the change, the most simple automatic and effortless activity of the skeleton becomes laboured and requires more energy. Subtle strains are stored up, and this means trouble. In its perfect functioning order, which is rare in reality, properly balanced muscle groups at the front, back and either side of the spine prevent it from deviating from a good alignment. Correct spinal alignment in turn places all the other joints in their best working positions.

But, sadly, too often in real life, because of our tendency to lead a sedentary life, routinely engaging in activities with a flexed or bent-over posture, the muscle groups which hold the skeleton upright become unevenly matched. Without our being aware of it, one group becomes tight and shorter while the opposing muscle group becomes weak and elongated. As a result, the upright skeleton is inadequately supported, out of trim with all its actions out of kilter. Everywhere joints are afflicted by poor working conditions; they are forced to work at awkward angles. They start to grind and chafe, and they are on the road to wearing out.

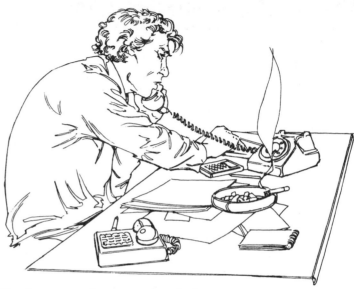

1 Much of our lives is spent like this, crumpled over in concentration with the joints bent.

Furthermore, because the skeleton becomes permanently kinked and constricted, we find we are at liberty to perform fewer and fewer movements. All purposeful activity takes place within a limited selection of available starting postures. We do not have the 'release' to do as we please with our bodies. We are trapped as if the wind has changed. Movements become stereotyped and repetitive, rarely introducing us to the benefit of full opening-out stretch. In fact we are most times unaware of the delights of full elastic freedom. Instead we tend to toil away within the same limited old patterns of movement. We put the toothbrush away, we open the car door; we might even go the whole day without doing one original movement. Day after day we grind the joints back and forth over the same old territory, never stretching them out into their other, forgotten directions. They joints lose their 'play' and become almost rigid except in their well-worn tracks. I don't have to tell you that this is not good for them.

With this background of imbalance, the working spine is debilitated in all the activities it carries out, all day and every day. Robbed of generous vital activity, the muscles and ligaments lose their bounce and the joints dry out and lose their slip. The final straw is when we *do* decide to get up out of that chair and do a bit of exercise. Unfortunately, we do it with such ferocious gusto that we introduce a whole lot of new and sudden strains on top of the old and subtle ones. The combination is a lethal one. No wonder 95 per cent of the population has or has had backache.

Mind you, there is a good reason why we are gripped by a sudden desire to leap out of that chair and fling ourselves into such frenzied activity in the name of sport. It is a subconscious attempt to redress the balance. It is an itching to experience a brief taste of the skeleton at full stretch. It makes us feel so good to open out the frame widely and sample the delights of extension rather than permanent static flexion. Sport is the modern-day method of release of energies hitherto used in foraging for food and fighting off enemies but sport stresses a handicapped skeleton. But, whether you engage in aggressive sport or not, if you lead a sedentary life sitting for hours behind a desk or hunched over a steering-wheel, unfortunately, with unnerving ease you will eventually 'do something' which hurts a joint in the spine. You then develop a simple linkage problem within the spine and this is the start. Sooner or later it will result in the appearance of pain. The pain may be a nuisance or a nightmare but, if the function fault worsens, the pain will intensify.

If we are to rectify the problem and thus get rid of the pain, we cannot afford to ignore the fact that the spine is failing to work properly. It is useless to swallow pills or strap yourself into a corset. It is often equally inappropriate to operate on the link surgically and try to fix things that way: rather like taking a hammer and chisel to a rusty door-hinge when really all it needs is a bit of oil. A scalpel cannot cut out stiffness, any more than a chisel can cut out rust. There is no object to be removed; the problem is a function fault.

By and large the cure for an aching back lies in persuading a stiff and painful spinal link to work better. Simply that. And here is the good news. The more the hinge is moved, the more it will want to move. It will self-lubricate as it is made to move back and forth and it will gradually stretch itself free of its stiffness. The pain disappears. I and all the other practitioners who work in the field of manual medicine, different as our individual approaches may be, have thousands upon thousands of patients who will testify to this. It works! This is what 'spinal mobilisation' and the rest of this book are all about.

2

BACK TO BASICS

WHAT IS A BACK?

The spine is a tall graceful column which rises out of the pelvis and waves in the breeze. It is jointed throughout its length into twenty-four small segments of bone called vertebrae.

Seven vertebrae make up the neck. Twelve vertebrae make up the thorax or the chest part of the spine. Each of these thoracic (or dorsal) vertebrae has a rib coming off either side which circles around the chest wall and joins up with the sternum, or breastbone, at the front. The ribs move as we breathe in, rather like bucket handles. With each in-breath, the ribs lift up and out as the lungs fill up with fresh air. As we breathe out and expel stale air, the bucket handles move down and in, as if to rest on the rim of the bucket until the next inspiration.

By and large the thoracic part of the spine moves less generously than any other part of the spine. This is hardly surprising when one considers the engineering feat in attaching a pair of ribs on either side of each vertebra of the thoracic spine. The ribs move incessantly every time we take a breath, and carry on doing this without faltering while at the same time that thoracic spine might be contorted into throwing a cricket ball or walking along talking to a colleague beside you or just bending over, doing up the shoe-laces.

Five vertebrae make up the low back part of the spine, sometimes called the lumbar spine, and this is the part of the spine I am going to talk about in this book. The lumbar vertebrae are very bulky and strong, built to carry a lot of weight but they are also exceedingly light. This is because the bones themselves are not solid. If you were to cut one open you would find it looks like honeycomb inside. In reality it is a three-dimensional grid of narrow bony pillars. Vertical ones act like struts which resist the flattening press-

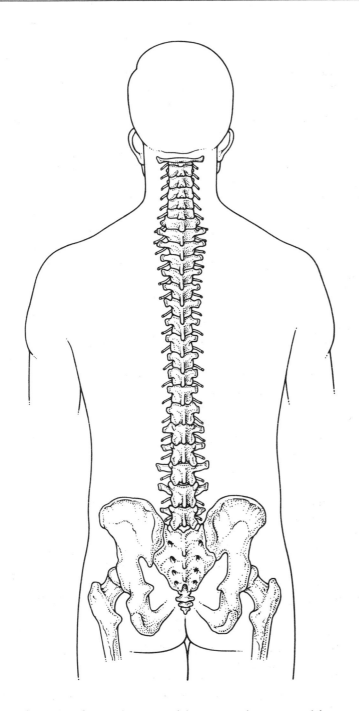

2 Posterior view of the human spine.

ure of weight from above and horizontal ones act like cross-bars which prevent the vertical ones from buckling. The lowest lumbar vertebra ends higher up in the body than you would think, on average about five centimetres below waist level.

The base of the spine joins on to the sacrum. This is a flat triangular wedge of bone which joins the two ear-shaped bones of the pelvis (the ilia) at the two sacro-iliac joints on either side where the two dimples can be seen on the surface at low-back level. The sacrum can be felt as a broad flat bone above the buttocks and it is made up of five fused sacral vertebrae. By 'fused' I mean they are permanently joined together and do not move, except in a congenital condition known as lumbarisation where the first sacral vertebra is mobile (see 'Have I an Extra Vertebra?' Chapter 3).

The coccyx projects off the tip of the sacrum as a brittle extension. It is the vestigial remnant of the tail. If it protrudes down too far, it can be bent under with a hard fall on to the bottom or bent backwards during childbirth as the baby is pushed out of the pelvis.

In its upright state, a normal spine carries itself with all the vertebrae stacked vertically in three gently arching curves perfectly designed to disperse the body weight in a balanced and effortless way. The lumbar spine hollows in slightly and the curve is called the lumbar lordosis; the thorax arches out slightly and the curve is called the thoracic kyphosis; and the neck arches in again in the cervical lordosis.

Each vertebra is separated from the next by beautifully designed little cushions of elastic tissue called the intervertebral discs. They consist of a soft squashy centre like a liquid pearl, called the nucleus, contained by a tough rim of concentric rings of fibrous tissue — the annulus. The annulus hold the nucleus tightly corseted in the centre of the disc. Discs are perfectly engineered to bear weight by acting as 'hydraulic sacks' and dispersing the pressure of the weight of the body above.

It is worth dwelling upon this upright stacking arrangement of the human spine, because there is an absurd popular belief that we are not designed to walk upright at all. Hearsay tells us that it is a bad arrangement and we really should be crawling about on all fours rather than striding about on two. This old wives' tale is one of the many which clutters the understanding of backs and shrouds the possibility of cure with an air of hopelessness and defeat.

I feel it is a great strain for a mobile column to be slung horizontally between widely separated front and back legs. Four-legged creatures must accept marked limitation in their functional performance because of this. A human being can get away with being relatively unfit and yet maintain itself in more or less upright posture. Any four-legged creature must be permanently fit, young and strong to prevent its spine sagging towards the floor just as it stands there. Overweight dachshunds, which have a long-drawn-out sausage-shaped body, commonly suffer from backache.

A superior co-ordination and balance mechanism, in combination with an upright spine, makes it possible for us to perform many more sophisticated activities than any other animals can do. The human spine has evolved in such a way that it can easily manage the different stresses. A horse can only go forwards either quickly or slowly. It could never pole-vault or stand on one leg. And who said horses never get backache? There is a whole stable of equine osteopaths out there who spend all their waking hours treating horses for ricked backs, especially the ones that jump fences. And those same horses might not yet be four years old! No, by and large, a spine is far better off working vertically than horizontally. There may be the occasional ballooning or even a blow-out of the wall of a disc lower down the spine where they are subjected to more weight (the 'slipped disc'), which may cause some trouble, but this is an uncommon cause of very common backache.

The human spine performs three basic functions. It provides *support* to keep us upright. It has the *mobility* to put two long arms out to handle, lift and push things; it adapts the torso to the walking process performed by the legs; it carries an extremely heavy head which constantly nods and swivels in the course of its functions. The spine therefore provides dynamic mobility and support. It also acts as *casing* to protect the valuable and fragile spinal cord, part of the central nervous system, which runs down the inside of the spinal column from the base of the brain. Spinal nerves which branch off from the cord pass out of the spinal casing at each intervertebral joint level. They leave the spine through short bony canals called intervertebral foraminae. These canals are created where two notches of two adjacent vertebrae come together making a bony gutter.

So it is true that those small sensitive nerves, almost as soon as they have branched off the mother cord, go straight into the jaws of the hinge between one bone and the next, to leave the spine. Not a good arrangement. That hinge only needs to get jammed or a bit rusty and watch out for that nerve!

This crucial combination where a delicate and important network of nervous pathways is so intimately related to a generously mobile mechanical structure can lead to trouble. It is a mechanical set-up which of necessity must be in perfect working order, because nervous tissue is extremely sen-

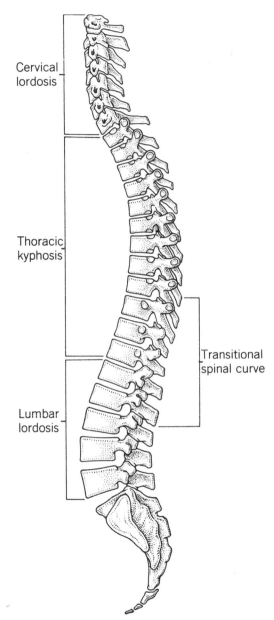

Cervical lordosis

Thoracic kyphosis

Transitional spinal curve

Lumbar lordosis

3 The human spine comprises seven cervical vertebrae, twelve thoracic and five lumber vertebrae.

23

4 The front vertebra-disc-vertebra compartment bears most of the weight, while the interlocking facet joints of the back compartment bear little weight but 'guide' the movement. The spinal nerve runs between the two.

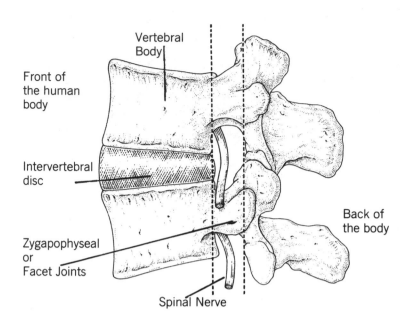

sitive and does not take kindly to being interfered with.

Imagine a healthy spine and its normal joints and you will see how easy it is for things to go wrong. If the mechanics of a spine go adrift, then pain is never far behind. The spinal joints at each intervertebral segment consist of a front and back compartment with the spinal canal containing the cord between. The front compartment consists of the vertebra-disc-vertebra joint. The disc adheres strongly to the body of the vertebra above and below. So as well as the vital role of bearing weight this complex also allows very strong and secure multidirectional movement of one vertebra on top of the other.

The disc-to-bone union is strengthened by the extremely strong anterior and posterior longitudinal ligaments. The anterior longitudinal ligament covers the front and sides of the round vertebral bodies; the posterior longitudinal ligament runs down the back of the vertebral bodies, and by covering the back wall of the discs it intercedes between the discs and the valuable nervous matter behind, lying in the spinal canal. Strong encircling ligament therefore runs down the entire length of the spine, encasing the round vertebral bodies in a strong elastic strait-jacket which controls movement.

Behind the spinal canal is the back compartment of the spinal joint, the apophyseal or facet joints. These joints are a simple bone-to-bone junction of neighbouring vertebrae.

Slippery glistening material called cartilage covers the two opposing bones and helps them to slide easily one against the other. Further friction is prevented by the presence of natural lubrication 'oil' called synovial fluid. The two opposite bones making up the joint are held in place by ligaments and the joint capsule, the inner lining of which manufactures the lubricating synovial fluid.

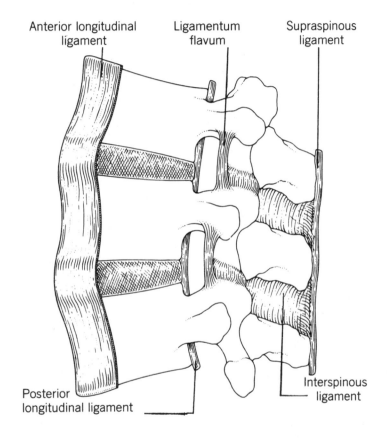

Anterior longitudinal ligament

Ligamentum flavum

Supraspinous ligament

Posterior longitudinal ligament

Interspinous ligament

5 The spinal ligaments.

The facet joints act as a bony 'catch' which helps to prevent one vertebra slipping off another. Their role therefore is to guide or stabilise the generous movement of the vertebra-disc compartment so that it does not become excessive. The facet joints act rather like the two little outrigger canoes stabilising the big canoe in the middle.

In a well-aligned lumbar spine these joints do not bear a lot of weight. However, when a back stands or sits with a deep hollow in the low lumbar area — an increased lumbar lordosis — these joints are forced to carry some weight. It is not what they were designed to do and they will complain.

WHY SHOULD A BACK GO WRONG?

The human spine can be likened to a ship's mast. It has 'stays' at the front, back and sides to provide a balanced support. In the case of the spine the stays are the balanced strength of the tummy muscles at the sides and front and the back muscles behind. Laxity in one of the stays will result in the mast either bowing forwards in the case of a slack front stay (weak tummy muscles) and an over-tight back stay (back muscles), or the mast bowing backwards if the front stay is too tight and the back stay is too long. The same happens if the back (stay) muscles are too weak.

Balanced opposing muscle groups of equivalent length and strength convert the torso into a mobile flexible cylinder, secure and confident in its work and well able to uphold the integrity of the brittle spinal column it protects. Unlike a ship's mast, however, the spine is jointed throughout its length into small segments. A complex neuro-muscular mechanism controls the movement of these segments all stacked on top of one another like a wobbling column of bricks.

The joints of the spine, like all other joints, have their movement controlled by muscles. Muscles work by contracting and shortening in their length and thus exerting leverage on the bones across a joint. Each muscle group always has an opposing group to make sure that all joint movement is balanced. It should be just as easy to get out of a movement as it was to do it in the first place. It would be very inconvenient, for example, if we could happily bend the elbow using the biceps but had no opposing group (triceps) to straighten it out again when we had finished using the arm in the bent position. It would be very clumsy indeed if we had to wait for the weight of the arm to pull the arm out straight again.

A sophisticated machinery for co-ordinating muscle activity acts all the time as we move, so that as one muscle group contracts (say, the biceps) the opposite muscle group (triceps) pays out or lets go at a perfectly regulated rate, so that the movement of the elbow is smooth and controlled and useful rather than jerky.

Usually, this co-ordination machinery works without a hitch and all joint action is controlled. However, every now and again we do something awkwardly or suddenly and jolt

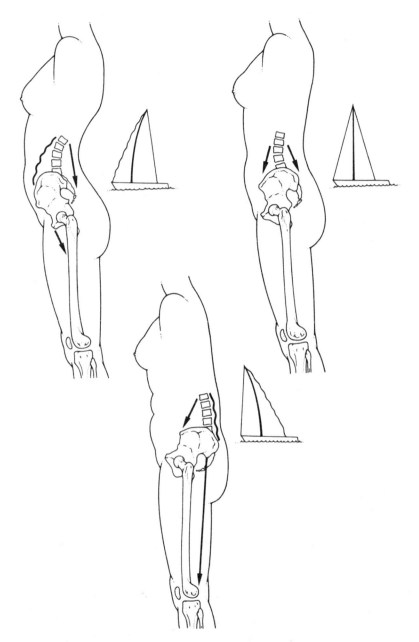

6 The effect on the spine when
there is a weakness of the stays
which stabilise the column.

the spine, catching the co-ordination machinery unawares.
The academics call it an 'interference of the co-relaxation
phenomenon'. The vigilant balanced interaction of the various muscle groups is caught off guard and we 'rick' the back.

Usually the spinal joints, like any other joint, can cope with this kind of shock. The shock-wave passes through the joint as a ripple or as a wrench. Because the joint is healthy and elastic, the two opposing bones making up the joint 'ride out' the distorting force by shuffling about a bit like boats riding at anchor. As the wave passes, they settle down again into their former loosely held harmony and there is minimal damage caused.

Sometimes, though, when such an event occurs one of the joints in this mobile and fluidly moving column may be strained. The reaction of living tissue to mechanical strains or sprains is always the same. If living tissue is hurt, it will weep. A mixture of blood and clear tissue fluid called lymph oozes out into the general area and creates the familiar puffiness of recent injury.

Joint strain can be trivial. There is a quick tug and release of the soft tissues binding the joint together and the fibres are stretched but not broken and there is minimal swelling. At the other extreme, there may be a massive tearing apart of the joint when most of the soft tissues are ripped and there is a pouring of blood and other fluid into the surrounding tissues with a lot of obvious swelling.

Depending on how much fluid escapes from the injured tissues, and depending on how much normal movement of the area was then possible to encourage that swelling to be pumped away and reabsorbed by the bloodstream, there will always remain a small residue of this fluid lying about the site of soft-tissue injury. Unfortunately, this creates problems. As the fluid lies there stagnating in the tissues, it dries out and goes hard. It also tends to shrink with age, and the effect is that the joint becomes confined by its own soft tissues and it loses mobility.

The natural legacy of straining a joint is that the joint will thereafter remain slightly stiff. In most cases you will not even be aware of this, and after a period of time normal activity and movement will work the joint free of this stiffness. It is much easier to strain your back if you are unfit, with some muscles weak and some muscles tight. The co-ordinated muscle control is slightly out of balance and less competent in its vigil against strain.

A joint mishap, as I said, may not necessarily be a major event. It may be felt as just a twinge which passes off immediately, or it may be a sickening searing pain through the back. However, once the joint is strained it remains strained. The spine stores the incident. The joint will go through a normal process of reaction. It will be inflamed and sore for a while. Then the soreness will pass and the joint will settle down again and become completely symptom-free. It will, however, remain slightly stiffer than it previously was and stiffer than its neighbours still are. This patch of stiffness is the core of the future back problem.

The stiff link remains. It need not be marked, just like a rusty link in a bicycle chain, or a sluggish key on the keyboard of a piano. For most of the time it happily participates with the rest of the spinal segments in functional activity — perhaps a bit more slothfully than its neighbours, but they will usually compensate for the patch of poor mobility by over-movement at the neighbouring joints. But the overall net movement of the spine will not be deficient. All goes well until it happens again: an awkward movement. It is more likely to happen again sooner if movement of the body generally has become distorted by the pain. The new awkward movement unavoidably demands participation of the spine exactly at the immobile joint. Because this segment is so stiff it is particularly vulnerable to strain. Being brittle and inelastic it cannot absorb the shock of the bad movement as it happens. The level that is already damaged and therefore handicapped suffers another strain because it is disabled.

The initial process of joint strain repeats itself, except that this time it is a little more dramatic with more inflammation caused. A few fibres may be torn as the joint is wrenched, and there may be swelling in and around the joints. If the joint is significantly irritated by the incident, the local spinal muscles may go into a reflex spasm in an attempt to protect the joint. The effect of the spasm is to hold the segment rigid to prevent as much movement as possible taking place there. The muscle spasm is painful in itself (as is any muscle when suffering low-grade cramp) and it may be felt as hard and uncomfortable cords of muscle either side of the spine like railway tracks. The spine becomes rigid and loses its gentle lumbar curve; doctors speak of loss of lumbar lordosis. When this happens, the trouble is fairly serious.

Sometimes, if you have not heeded the signals of discomfort and have continued to do too much, the muscle spasm will become even more overactive in an effort to protect the strained underlying joint. This has the effect of jamming the hurt joint together even more and disallowing any movement at all — that lovely therapeutic movement which it so badly needs in order to start mending itself. Conversely, the muscle spasm may become heightened if the patient does too little and lies about in bed too frightened to do anything

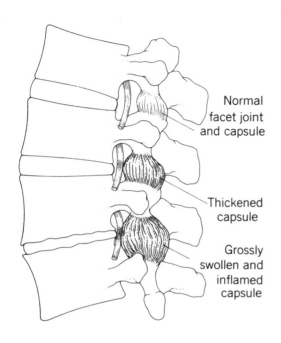

Normal
facet joint
and capsule

Thickened
capsule

Grossly
swollen and
inflamed
capsule

7 The progressive degeneration of a facet joint. As the disc shrinks there will be over-riding of the two joint surfaces and puckering of the swollen capsule.

with his back. The result will be the same, with the two bony surfaces staying jammed together with the joint getting more bloated and stiff because it is being denied the benefit of gentle movement — rhythmic gentle movement which gets the blood going and unleashes the healing process. Usually, guided by intuition and common sense, you will get going again at the right rate after minimal time spent lying about. The joint soreness settles, the muscle spasm dies away and the incident passes.

If the muscle spasm stays severe and persistent, over a period of time — and I believe very much as a secondary development to the previously described process — the degenerated intervertebral disc, having been squashed by the vice-like pressure of the muscles in spasm, will be pinched out between the two adjacent vertebrae; the so-called slipped disc. Bear in mind, too, that the fibrous wall of this disc may have been traumatised over the years by the incessant wear and tear of torsional strains which will have weakened the strong corset-like wall and rendered it more susceptible to bulging. But when and if the muscle spasm relaxes, the joint surfaces will start to jostle and move apart again as the whole segment begins to disimpact. The disc bulge will disappear as the muscle clamp comes off.

If this process of progressive stiffening of a link in the spine develops into a more serious complaint, the entire spine becomes disabled. Eventually you can do very little at all without stretching the stiff joint and provoking the muscles to clench even harder. The joint is therefore being continuously irritated by normal activity and permanent inflammation, and pain will be the result.

As a segment becomes less active the intervertebral disc separating the two vertebrae at the affected level will tend to shrivel — the collapsed disc — or, even more emotional, the disintegrating disc. It is easy to see why discs keep healthy as long as we keep moving well. Just as soon as we start to lose spinal mobility, the process of disc degeneration accelerates.

As the disc loses height, one vertebra tends to sink down on to the vertebra below. The bony catches at the back of the vertebral segment tend to override down on to each other and the working hinges of the spine become even more jammed.

It is possible that a joint may become completely impacted, with one vertebra almost completely fused to its neighbour below and very little disc between. This state of affairs may mean that all movement is completely obliterated at that level, and since nothing can budge the joint it is very hard to hurt it. The condition may be painless.

WHERE DOES THE PAIN COME FROM?

People specialising in the management of back pain have been slow to answer that question, perhaps because we ourselves have been confused. However, what we do know is that there is an enormous variation in the capacity of the different structures in the back to register pain. Some cry pain at the slightest provocation whereas other structures are much more hardy.

Discs barely have a nerve supply. Remember that point! Only the outermost rim of the annulus of the disc has pain-sensing nerve fibres. A disc therefore can only be held responsible for causing pain if it is in some way damaged at this point of supply. This only happens if there is a small strain of the fibres of a healthy disc wall, which is rare, or if the entire disc is in the most advanced stages of degeneration, which is not so rare. The latter usually accompanies a loss in disc height, revealed by X-ray. Irrespective of whether a disc wall is emitting pain or not, disc walls often bulge. They are meant to bulge — they are shock absorbers. But it is thought that the effects of this bulge rather than the bulge itself are the main genesis of pain. The bulge may press upon or squash other soft-tissue structures nearby, which are positively 'electrified' by a pain-sensitive nerve supply. Wired for pain.

Two structures liable to be squashed by an unwanted disc bulge are the posterior longitudinal ligament and the spinal nerve root. Irritation of the spinal nerve will be discussed in greater detail later in this chapter; for the moment we will discuss irritation of the posterior longitudinal ligament.

The posterior longitudinal ligament is extremely rich in nerve supply and very touchy whenever it is subjected to unusual mechanical stresses or to chemical irritation from nearby inflammation. And it is possible that an unhealthy bulging intervertebral disc can painfully stretch and distort the posterior longitudinal ligament. Then you will feel backpain.

Interestingly enough, the posterior ligament begins to

narrow in its width at the upper lumbar level, so that at the level of L.4 and L.5 (the vertebral levels most commonly afflicted by disc bulges) it is only half the width that it was higher up the spine. It could almost be said that this is a careful design detail, since it tapers in width as it nears the site of most common disc-bulge activity, thereby reducing its exposed flank to assault.

Other very sensitive structures inside a back, commonly responsible for sending out pain messages, are the facet joints. They are situated at the back of each individual spinal vertebra, two sets, top and bottom (see diagram 9).

These little joints have a very rich nervous network which keeps the brain constantly bombarded with information on how the joint is working. If the facet joints are malfunctioning, their own nerve supply will reveal this in the form of pain.

Trouble with the facet joints of the spine is the commonest cause of backpain. You only have to recall the astonishing versatility of this flexible column to realise that, although it is generous in its performance, it is vulnerable. Sudden or ill-considered movements can rick a joint. The joint swells and then goes stiff, becoming in itself an ample source of pain.

Think how distressingly painful a twisted ankle is. The joints of the back are no different from ankle joints except that they are much smaller and there are more of them crowded into a small space, with a dense network of sensitive nerves threading throughout. When an ankle starts to swell and creak on movement, we really know about it. Backpain is just the same — except that the back is less precise in telling us exactly where and what is hurting.

To make matters worse, in addition to the joint being swollen and painful, its excessively engorged bulk may press on, and hurt, the nearby spinal nerve. More pain. This time from both the joint and the nerve.

This brings me to the spinal nerves themselves, which are extremely pain-sensitive. They can be irritated chemically by noxious irritants resulting from inflammation nearby or they can be irritated by being physically squashed. It is not uncommon for a nearby disc or facet joint to malfunction thus causing them to swell. Unfortunately, because the nerve lies so close to these sites of trouble, it is itself directly irritated and raises the alarm of pain. And it is a pretty nasty type of pain, too. It is known as sciatica, or 'projected' nerve-root pain, and is particularly unpleasant. Typically described as 'lancinating', it shoots down the leg in a sharp searing wave

L.1.

Posterior
longitudinal
ligament

L.2.

L.3.

L.4.

L.5.

8 The pain-sensitive posterior longitudinal ligament is narrower over the L.4–L.5 and L.5–S.1 disc spaces where bulges are more common.

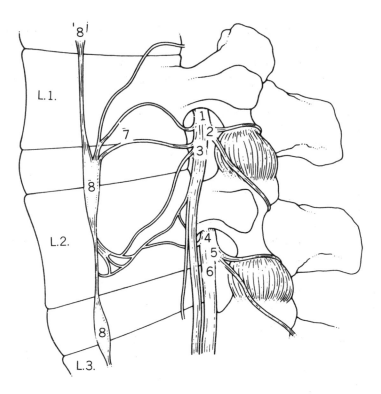

1 – 1st lumbar nerve
2 – Dorsal lumbar nerve
3 – Ventral lumbar nerve
4 – 2nd lumbar nerve
5 – Dorsal lumbar nerve
6 – Ventral lumbar nerve
7 – Rami communicans
8 – Sympathetic truck ganglion

9 All facet joints are clothed in a complex interlinking lace-work of nerves.

of agony. It is often associated with numbness, or pins and needles, or both.

Another spinal component which is less commonly the source of painful symptoms from the back is the dura, that thin film of membranous matter which wraps around and protects the spinal cord as it hangs down inside the spinal column (see 'Why is Sitting so Uncomfortable?' Chapter 9). Sometimes because of longstanding inflammation of one or more of the spinal segments, this membrane, too, becomes inflamed, simply as a result of its close proximity to the primary site of inflammation. The legacy of inflammation is the same here as it is with all other soft-tissue structures: the dura in effect shrinks and loses its ability to stretch. It does not take a lot of imagination to envisage, therefore, that a mobile spine tethered from within will be a problem one. On manual examination, the lumbar spine often feels puckered in or bunched up as if it were beads of a necklace threaded on to an elastic string which is too tight. Any postural position, especially one which puts the spine (and the dura) on a sustained stretch, will tug at the dura and cause pain. Dural pain is very diffuse. You would have a hard job pin-pointing exactly where in the back you feel pain. It

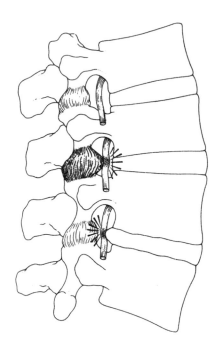

10 The delicate spinal nerve can be pinched either by a swollen disc or by a swollen facet joint capsule.

might extend up as far as the shoulder blades and around to the front of the abdomen. This phenomenon also accounts for the patient's startling though not uncommon testimony that a headache comes and goes as the low-back pain comes and goes.

Let us stop at this point to dwell on one very important fact: there are only a few structures in a back which can be painful. Mysterious, even frightening, as backpain might be, the cause may be quite simple. More significantly, pain will always be associated with an abnormality of local spinal performance. In this way it is possible for an 'outsider' like me to know where a back will be painful. It always corresponds to the part of the spine which is not moving properly.

In fact it is very easy for a therapist to feel (with the hands) whether an area of the spine is not functioning properly. It takes a bit more assessment and examination to deduce which structure in particular is causing the movement anomaly and therefore needs some therapeutic attention. For example, it is not so easy to tell if the problem is primarily a disc problem or primarily a facet joint problem, because, although we can feel the facet joints, we cannot feel the discs. It may be an oversimplification, but as a rule I only consider that a back problem might be discogenic if there is no abnormality in the feel of the facet joints.

Problem lumbar facet joints are easy to feel. We examine the joints of the low back by lying you face down, comfortable and relaxed on the couch with a pillow under the tummy to slacken off the lumbar spine completely. By probing deep into the back with the thumbs, about two and a half centimetres either side of the spinal knobs, one can feel these joints. They can barely be felt in their healthy state. They willingly slide away under the pressure of the approaching thumbs and are conspicuous only by their inconspicuousness.

In their pain-making state, however, the facet joints feel quite different in a variety of ways. They are always enlarged or swollen. They may also have a hard brittle feel, so that the joint, clothed in its capsule and its ligaments, feels exactly like a tough little ping-pong ball — indicating, by the way, an older, 'drier' joint problem. Or there may be a softer, tense but squashy feel rather like a half deflated squash-ball, which indicates a more recent problem.

If there has been a poorly functioning segment in the spine for some time, the general state of the tissues around that joint will be thickened and leathery. On the first cursory feel of the back, simply running the fingers down the spine, the problem areas are immediately apparent to the therapist, even before the joints themselves are felt.

A disc is impossible to feel because it is right around the front of the spine, far out of reach of the fingers, so that the actual bulging wall of a problem disc is not directly helped by manually moving (mobilising) the vertebrae. However, we do get results with disc problems, using mobilisation. We think that the benefit is derived from gentle loosening of the uppermost segment, which shakes it free of its impaction to the one below. By increasing mobility at that lumbar level we help gently to 'lift' the top impacted vertebra off the bottom one, thus taking the pressure off the bulge.

Problem discs, then, are only indirectly helped by manual intervention of the thumbs into the back, but swollen and painful facet joints are another story altogether when it comes to the laying on of hands! The weary back sufferer, ensnared for years in a solitary struggle with pain, will experience a profound sense of comfort and relief when he feels, for the first time, the sure and knowing touch of experienced hands. From my point of view, it can be gratifying to observe. Not infrequently I feel an immense outpouring of compassion for a beleaguered patient, so beaten by pain.

11 It is easy to feel the facet joints.

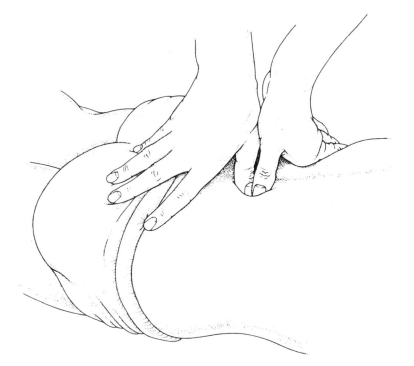

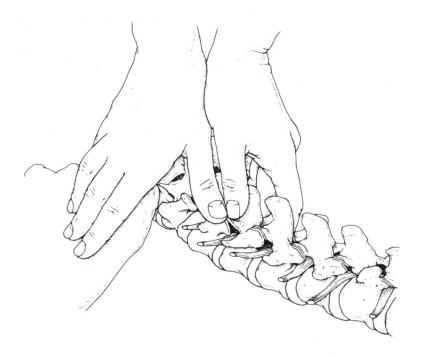

Meek and obedient, we are all children when locked in the jaws of pain. Time and time again, without demur, these desperate people will unquestioningly offer up their wretched backs for us to have a go at. It is not difficult to see how shamefully easy it is for such people to fall into the hands of the unscrupulous practitioner who will promise the world and abuse a sore spine sickeningly to achieve that end.

But human touch is a neglected balm; more is the pity, because it can be powerful medicine, so deft and sure that it seems almost magical. Furthermore, thumbs are perfectly designed to delve around in the human spine.

3

DIAGNOSING THE PROBLEM

Apart from their backs, back sufferers always have two complaints: one, that everyone is bored and possibly disbelieving about the problem and, two, that they are never exactly told what is wrong.

In truth, it is hard to be sure what exactly is wrong. The spine is an extremely sophisticated piece of machinery and in all probability, if you have been having trouble for some time, there will be more than one thing wrong.

Without wishing to seem pedantic, there is no option but to make a thoughtful guess. Patients expect to be told. One has to make a stab at replying to their imploring questions. It is half of the job.

Every day I am asked the same sorts of questions. You patients are very interested in what is wrong with you. I know at times you think of very little else. But bear in mind that answers are only informed assumptions and one can never speak in absolute terms. Medicine is not an exact science; there are too many humans involved in it.

HAVE I SLIPPED A DISC?

Disc trouble is not as common as everyone thinks, but when it does occur it is the most difficult back problem to manage conservatively. Ultimately the problem disc will need to be surgically removed.

To describe what goes wrong with a disc, I must first of all describe a normal disc.

Our discs dampen the shock of spinal movement. They are resilient little fibro-elastic cushions that sit between the vertebrae and cushion the bone-to-bone junction. Each disc is strongly adherent to the bottom of the vertebra above and the top of the vertebra below. At the centre of the disc is a liquid ball-bearing or spherical fluid nucleus which acts as a hydraulic sack and disperses the heavy weight of the body bearing down upon it. The nuclear material is jelly-like in nature and exhibits a unique ability to attract water to itself. This helps partially to ensure that liquid remains in the centre of the disc when it is subjected to compressive forces. Furthermore, the high water content of the nucleus transmits load to the periphery, either in an upward direction, which tends to counter the super-incumbent weight, or in a radial or outward thrust, which reduces the tendency for the outer wall of the disc to buckle under the heavy load.

The outer wall of the disc (the annulus) is unusually strong but it is also elastic. It is made up of concentric rings of fibrous material, meshed together to make a thick rim. Each successive layer of meshed wall has fibrous strands aligned at 90 degrees to those of the adjacent layer, making a living lattice just like the walls of a radial car-tyre. The incompressible make-up of the lattice makes the discs unsquashable, like high-tensile springs.

This combination of high-tensile elastic walls and a powerfully self-centred jelly sack in the middle of the disc is a tenaciously stable arrangement. This means that the nucleus cannot be forced, under pressure, out of the centre of the disc if the disc is in its normal healthy state. Even experimentally creating a radial cut in the wall of a disc with a scalpel blade will not result in the nucleus squeezing out through the slit. This in itself disproves the widely held notion that one ill-considered movement can 'put a disc out'. Nuclear material only squashes out when it has degenerated or degraded. But more about that later.

The properties of a mobile ball-bearing centre and a very strong disc-retaining wall make possible the spectacular mobility of the spine. They allow each vertebra to sit on top of its neighbour below and roll around confidently in secure and grandiose spinal movement.

These discs unfortunately are wont to degenerate and in this diseased state may cause trouble. As described earlier, in the aftermath of a previous jolt or wrench to the spine, a vertebral segment may unobtrusively tighten up and become less mobile. This has unfortunate consequences for the disc, since it relies to a great degree on full segmental movement to suck in fluid and food. The lack of movement deprives it of fluid exchange and as a result it will silently starve, causing it to lose vitality. The shrinkage of the nucleus at the

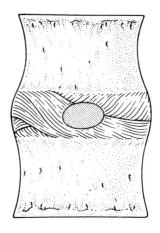

12.1 The wall of the disc is like a living lattice.

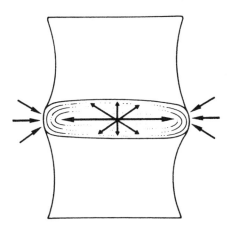

12.2 The disc as a hydraulic sack dispersing pressure.

centre of the disc places an extra load on the rim or wall, where radial splits begin to appear as a result of wear and tear. Pushed along particularly by repetitive bending and twisting movements of the body, the nucleus soon takes this exit route from the centre of the disc.

Another mode of degeneration of the disc has recently been described by Twomey and Bogduk, two leading Australian researchers in the biodynamics of the lumbar spine. They postulate that the first stage of the process is a fracture of the end-plate, the flat bone surface of the vertebrae immediately adjacent to the disc. This is the weakest point in the internal make-up of the spine, particularly if it is vertically compressed. The impaction caused by a heavy fall onto the bottom say, can cause the bone to 'cave in'. This is a fairly serious injury, in which it is thought that part of the nucleus is forced into the broken cavity of bone. Here it comes into contact with the blood stream where it is seen as 'foreign matter' and the auto-immune defences of the body are activated. The disc gradually degrades. As it deflates the wall or rim bears a greater brunt of the load. The nucleus loses its ability to hold water and is rendered 'expressible' or able to be pushed out of the centre of the disc.

If, by chance, there is a radial split close by, the result of accelerating trauma to the disc wall, it is easy to see how the unhealthy material can squirt out through the crack. Forward bending and twisting movements of the body can cause the crack to open up more which explains why it is often these very movements which ultimately cause the disc to 'go' — the last straw.

However, whatever the reasons for the gradual deterioration of internal disc health, usually the nuclear material does not burst right through the disc wall (the herniated disc). More commonly it only squeezes part of the way through the multiple layers of wall. But the build-up of pressure in front of the 'straying' nucleus severely distends the few layers of wall which remain intact, and you get your bulge (the slipped or protruding disc).

This can cause a squashing of other pain-sensitive structures close by, the most sensitive of which is the spinal nerve root. But as stated earlier, the notion of 'the slipped disc pinching a nerve' is undergoing some scrutiny. It has long been acknowledged that pressure alone upon nerves situated in other parts of the body does not cause pain. The funny-bone, for example, is a point at the elbow where the ulnar nerve is vulnerable to pressure. But if you hit the funny-bone or more likely squash it by lying awkwardly on

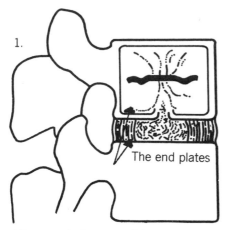

1.

Microscopic fracture of the
body of vertebra causes
the nucleus to degrade

The end plates

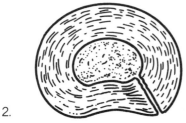

2.

Radial split from 'pinching'
with wear and tear allows
the nucleus an exit route

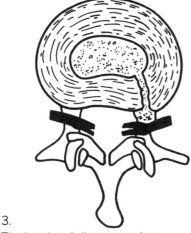

3.

The herniated disc pressurises
and inflames the spinal
nerve root

13 The story of disc degeneration.

your arm, you will feel only numbness and pins and needles, admittedly an unpleasant sensation, but never pain.

It is now thought that disc bulges alone do not worry the nearby pain sensitive structures in the back unless that pressure creates inflammation – redness, soreness, oozing and swelling. And then you will have trouble. The posterior longitudinal ligament is another nearby structure which inflames under pressure. Irritation of it and the spinal nerve can give you either back or leg pain or both.

Left unchecked, a disc problem often generates wider spinal disharmony which can feed back and worsen the original disc complaint. Complications set in as the disc loses height. The sudden loss of stature leads to local jamming of the link, which in turn disrupts over-all spinal movement. The muscles beside the spine go into a heightened state of contraction, or *spasm*, and an increasingly tense and bulging wall of disc is squeezed out. The spasm is simply an automatic protective mechanism which locks up the problem link, but it rapidly turns a nuisance state into a serious one. The pressure within the locked link is great and the inflammation rises to a crescendo. As the back grows tighter, more pressure is exerted on the sick link, the disc gets more squashed, its wall bulges further and the local engorgement and inflammation intensifies. And you may be completely incapacitated by a crippling pain in the leg — sciatica. If you lie low for a bit, the inflammation will slowly die away. But when the fire goes out, the affected segment may take on a totally different character. Though it is not 'hot' any more, the segment may become unstable. This happens because the impaction of the joint leaves the soft tissues which surround it and bind it together, in a lengthened, slack state. They become unable to hold the joint together because the opposing surfaces have settled closer together, deprived of a thick juicy wedge of normal disc to keep it tightly sprung apart. As the hot episode cools and the protective muscle spasm subsides, at least the tissues are decompressed which eases the inflammation, but the weak link is exposed, vulnerable again, for the cycle to repeat. It starts to slip around with normal movement which further stretches the binding ligaments. The tissues are irritated by the instability and it starts to hot up again.

All in all, the back behaves in a very unstable manner, causing the patient great anxiety, particularly about the possibility of having to submit to surgery. There will be increasingly frequent flare-ups with shorter respites between, and the incidents which set off an attack will increasingly trivial. The back will feel like a piece of board, stiff and sore for most of the time but interspersed with unnerving episodes when it suddenly 'gives way' and folds up at the weak link. Even the simplest tasks become chores. Spontaneity of movement is lost. It is hard to say exactly how the disc behaves but I suspect it fluctuates between phases of flaccidity and angry distension; 'good days and bad', as patients often say.

You find you can get by most of the time with a fairly rigid back as long as you don't sit for too long but you will be exasperated and wary of this rotten piece of machinery called your back. This makes 'tricky' backs very hard to treat by manual management and they usually need a laminectomy and spinal fusion (see 'Do I Need an Operation?' Chapter 4).

As the disc deteriorates, the nuclear material sometimes actually bursts through its retaining wall. When the pressure escapes, at least the squashed neighbouring soft tissues are decompressed, but it is thought that the nuclear material, by now well degenerated and a typical brownish colour, is itself a noxious irritant which inflames the surrounding tissues, providing an additional source of pain.

In either case the pain would be considerable, either in the back or the leg or both. Being loath to stand on the bad leg, you would tend to stand with the bad knee bent, a rounded low back often with an 'S' bend of the spine (the result of unequal contraction of the paired muscles on either side of the spine) with one hip-bone protruding prominently. It would be extremely difficult to sit or to move about and if forced to make a journey — for example, to see the doctor or have an X-ray — you may even be forced to lie down on the pavement or the floor to gain relief when the pain becomes intolerable. You may have difficulty passing urine and you may also experience numbness and/or muscle weakness in the leg. The only solution is for a surgeon to decompress the area by removing the disc (and some of the nearby bone, to achieve maximum decompression). Usually the results of such surgery are spectacularly good and the patient will awake from the anaesthetic with none of that awful pain.

Another disorder in the news these days is 'primary disc disease'. This diagnosis recognises that a sick disc alone can be a source of pain, irrespective of whether it is bulging (slipped) or not. The disc's health might have been sabotaged in the past by a microscopic traumatic fracture of the

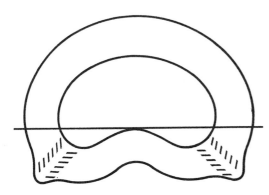

The disk wall
is pinched by rotatory
movements which
causes radial splits

*14 The typical sites of greatest wear
and tear are in the left and right
hand back corners of the disc
wall.*

end-plate as mentioned above — the result of a bad fall or a heavy blow — and this starts the nucleus degrading. As a result, undue strain, more like ligament strain, is suffered by the wall of the disc and this leads to pain.

Clinically, the diagnosis of primary disc disease isn't easy. You have to rely heavily on MRI scanning (a black disc on MRI means the disc is sick). Discs afflicted by primary disc disease often go on to bulge if the wall develops cracks through further wear and tear, whereafter you might get leg pain as well as the original back pain. But you can also preempt this with the proper management. These backs aren't easy to treat. I find them some of the hardest cases, not least because months might go by when progress seems assured, only to have a discouraging setback for no reason at all. They flare up with amazing capriciousness with the back stiffening and assuming the characteristic 'S' bend. Sitting seems to be the worst. The lack of pressure within the disc appears to make the spine 'slew around' on the problem disc like a car slewing around on a half-flat tyre. The disc walls traumatise and the pain signals go out.

Mobilisation can help to some extent which I explain by the manual tinkering injecting some looseness into the tightly held segment and hopefully relieving the squashing of the disc and distension of the wall. But perhaps greatest benefit is achieved through tummy exercises. They will shore up the spine within the torso, to reduce the burden carried by the slewing disc. The increased intra-abdominal pressure created by sit-up exercises, thrusts the spine skywards, just like squeezing a toothpaste tube with the cap screwed on. As the grip tightens, the tube will force itself upright. In the case of the spine, the greater the up-thrust, the more it lifts off itself and lesser the load borne by the sick disc.

If this back would seem to be you, then I suggest you read the section on exercises (see 'What Exercises Should I Do?' Chapter 6). It is essential for your welfare. A tight torso is your future. In that section I've deliberately emphasised the difference between good sit-ups and bad sit-ups. Your aim should be to curl up as you crease or fold the trunk across the middle. Try not to jerk up with a hollow in the low back. This action mainly uses the powerful hip muscles which will inhibit effective use of the pure abdominals group and it will unfavourably impact the lower lumbar vertebrae.

HAVE I PUT MY BACK OUT?

As a practitioner dealing almost solely with problem backs, I could not count the number of patients who have presented themselves to me with: 'I've put my back out.'

The automatic defence mechanisms which guard our posture and our balance are far too efficient to allow a spinal segment to dislocate completely during the course of simple everyday activity. The discs are strongly attached to the two vertebrae between which they sit and therefore cannot be dislodged with movement; the term 'slipped disc' is an absurdly inaccurate expression.

However, it is possible that one joint in the long chain of facet joints up either side of the spine can slip a tiny bit askew with a chance awkward movement. It is thought that a minor slip of a millimetre or two (called a subluxation) can manage to take place without the postural defences registering in time. Too late the spinal muscles react to stop the slip and they contract with one massive spasm. This may jam the two congruent surfaces of the joint, but jam them slightly out of alignment. This is known as 'facet locking', but it is a rare course of events.

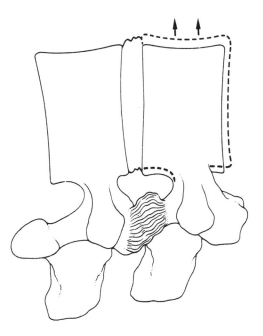

15 *Spinal instability is a common sequel to degeneration of both facet joint and intervertebral disc.*

The circumstance which leads to the facet joint becoming wobbly and likely to slip askew in the first place is incipient degeneration of the interceding disc, as described above. This creates a loose link in the spinal chain, because as the disc degenerates it loses water content and therefore height, like a hot-water bottle losing water. The segment becomes sloppy because it is no longer sprung apart by a thick, healthy disc. This type of back problem is distinguishable from the syndrome described previously ('Have I Slipped a Disc?') because in this facet-locking instance the disc has no role to play. It has simply shrunk and withered away leaving the facet joints to play out the scenario of dysfunction.

The capsule and the other soft tissues binding the facet joint together may become slack and unable to control fine movement of the vertebrae. They are then solely dependent on vigilant muscle control to prevent any untoward movement taking place. Alas! this is quite a tall order and often they cannot prevent you jarring the joint with the most trivial and incidental movement: for example, avoiding someone approaching you on the footpath or stepping off a deeper kerb than you had expected. Both may give you an agonising jab of pain. This is because the muscles were caught off guard and failed to brace you (but, more particularly, the sloppy joint) for the shock.

Sometimes the whole segment gets sloppier and sloppier because of incompetent ligament binding and it is said to be 'hyper-mobile'. If this happens, it is possible repeatedly to put the back out with increasing frequency and by more and more trivial means. Some of the more common precipitating incidents are sneezing, turning over in bed, getting up out of a chair or car — but the list is endless. One woman did it zipping up her ball dress.

However, you might present yourself for treatment saying that the back feels disjointed, as if it needs to be 'put back in'. Almost invariably it hasn't been put out in the manner I have just described. Usually it is simply that a joint had been stressed and is now locked up by protective muscles. It is now not working properly and causes the characteristic 'catching' pain as the muscles 'grab' whenever the joint is further threatened by a worrying movement.

The two different circumstances are easily distinguishable from one another. The acute subluxation takes place with a tweak or a cracking sound, followed almost instantaneously by a violent muscle spasm which completely takes your breath away and may even bring you to the floor. You become stuck in the movement as if frozen in time.

On the other hand, the incident of the joint strain can almost take place without you being aware of it. Characteristically, you will gradually develop a stiff back the night after chopping wood or painting the ceiling. You have not put anything 'out' — neither the joint nor the disc. But the trouble with the joint strain problem is that it suffers from the lack of a suitably colourful and descriptive catchphrase to describe it. It means nothing when you say to your friends that you have a poorly functioning joint in your spine and you must hurry off to see your physiotherapist to put it right. But if you say you have put your back out they are full of sympathy.

The best treatment approach for this joint strain injury is gently to persuade the poor defensive joint in its state of great alarm that movement is not such a bad thing after all and that movement is what it needs — gentle mobilisation with the thumbs, not another quick yank with a manipulation!

However, the facet locking or jamming is best dealt with by a quick manipulative thrust. This will momentarily 'spring' the joint apart and let it close back together again, properly aligned with the two congruent joint surfaces happily notched together again.

A manipulative procedure with the characteristic 'cracking' sound has its single most satisfactory application in this instance. Unfortunately, the patient rarely gets to the physiotherapist soon enough, before severe protective muscle spasm has set in. And the muscle spasm precludes the use of a quick thrust in the correct direction because it will not allow any movement of the spine at all at the affected level. If this is the case, a good deal of time has to be spent relaxing the area and getting rid of the muscle spasm so that eventually it can be manipulated. This may take days, but the problem will not be cleared until it has been manipulated. However, if we are lucky and can get in quickly and manipulate, the patient who arrived at the treatment session bent over and locked in one position will walk away from the treatment as good as new.

As a routine practice, it is not a good idea repeatedly to manipulate a joint which has become sloppy because of degeneration of the disc. Although one quick delicate thrust may be necessary to unlock a localised jamming, any more than that will simply make the joint more and more stretched and weak with an increasing propensity to slip askew in the future. Although there may be an immediate advantage in freeing the joint, the net long-term effect on the joint is an undesirable one. It further stretches the structures which are trying so hard to hold the segment stable.

Indeed, it is in this way that patients get locked into a pattern where they are permanently having treatment. Their symptoms are real enough, but they are being propagated by the treatment. It is not unusual to hear of patients who have been having manipulation once a week for as long as they can remember. If there is any blame to be apportioned in this instance, some of it must rest with the patients themselves. There are many people who do not feel that they have had a good enough treatment if they have not been manipulated. Further, they are unwilling to submit to being mobilised instead because they feel it does not 'do enough'. Although the treatment of choice might be gently to free the joint with the thumbs and to follow that with some exercise to tighten up the segment, it may at first encounter feel very passive and namby-pamby. I have heard before now: 'She didn't seem to be doing anything, just pressing with her hands!' Well, all I can say is: Just give it a chance. The alternative may be permanent treatment using techniques that are keeping you in need of treatment.

DO I HAVE ARTHRITIS?

Poor Western man, he gets arthritis just as he sits there. With his predilection for the sedentary life in which so much functional activity is done hunched over in a stooped posture performing a series of tasks notable only by their lack of variety, he stores up a heap of trouble for himself. No wonder, because he develops a working skeleton regulated by muscle groups which are out of balance and are of dissimilar ability.

It would be better if we ran around throwing spears all day and squatted in front of camp-fires instead of slumping in easy chairs watching telly. As it is, the unequal pull of muscles across the joints amounts to permanent wear and tear on the joints; arthritis is creeping in. Even in our most inactive moments, it takes its toll. The joints do not work at their best when they are guided by disproportionate control.

Furthermore, joints that rarely enjoy the full excursion of their entire range of movement develop a reduced ability to carry out any movement that they do have. The joints develop reduced range of movement.

The great advantage about the living piece of machinery called the skeleton is that the more one demands movement of the joints, the better the joints respond and increase their self-lubrication. Movement keeps the joints fully mobile.

This fact alone makes it easy to see why therapy by movement is the only way! A stretchy, well-lubricated joint is a healthy one that never gives you any trouble (unless you injure it afresh with some other new incidental wrench or blow). So the less you move, the less you are able to; the more they dry out and deteriorate. 'Rest' for arthritis is not the answer.

Now, to explain that word 'arthritis' which worries everyone so! All of us, beyond teenage years, experience degenerative changes of various joints because, as I have said, of the limited ways we use our bodies. This speeds up the ageing of the joints. Then the joints are aged further by all the other incidental damaging jolts and bangs that any skeleton cannot help but suffer during everyday life.

These prematurely old joints are too tight for their own good and are extremely intolerant to shock. This is arthritis as we commonly know it. It is simply the normal ageing process of joints hurried along a bit by the knocks of life. It is not a 'disease'. It is simply wear and tear, and every joint will suffer it to a degree. Only in its more advanced form will it be a source of pain.

Nearly all the important joints of the body are known as synovial joints. They are joints as you would imagine them to be: two articulating bone-ends covered with cartilage, held together in a bag called a capsule, the sides of which are reinforced by ligaments. But synovial joints also provide their own fluid so that they can self-lubricate. Let us look at a synovial joint in its healthy state. This will make it easier to see what happens in its unhealthy state when it will give you pain.

The capsule is the 'sleeve' of soft tissue which binds the two bones of a joint together. The inner lining of the capsule is called the synovial membrane. The role of this membrane is to ooze fluid, called synovial fluid, which oils the bony machinery of the joint. Synovial fluid is magical stuff. Scientists have found it quite impossible to duplicate synthetically. A pity that some man-made oil cannot be squirted into all those painful and audibly squeaking joints to ease their troubled toil!

Synovial fluid exhibits the most astonishing qualities of lightness and slipperiness. This fluid, in combination with the shiny and smooth cartilage covering the two opposing bone surfaces, makes for quiet and effortless movement of two bones against one another in a joint.

The natural tension of the capsule and its synovial lining creates a hydraulic sack which in a normal healthy weight-bearing joint disperses the pressure of the weight through the joint by thrusting the two bones apart. This means, for example, in the case of the knee joint that we are not actually walking on the bones themselves and grinding them down. The bones barely even touch — they just sort of slip and slide over one another, sprung apart by the pressure of the fluid within the joint. The pressure within the joint is maintained by the natural tension of all ligaments and soft tissues holding the joint together. That is why a torn ligament of the knee creates such havoc. It is like a blow-out. The integrity of the knee has been fundamentally disturbed.

Normal efficient and effortless function of weight-bearing joints is further aided by the surprising plasticity of the bone underlying the cartilage. It can actually bend and absorb weight and other stresses more than you would think. Bone is actually very bendable.

Things start to deteriorate and the joints become 'arthritic' when the flow of fluid into the joint slows down to a trickle;

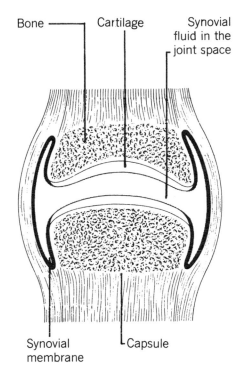

16 A normal synovial joint.

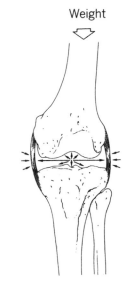

17 A normal joint acts like a hydraulic sack.

the cartilage and the bone become brittle and the other soft tissues — ligaments, tendons and muscles — dry out and lose their stretch. The bone loses its 'give and take' and the cartilage becomes damaged by acting as a buffer to the unyielding mass. The cartilage becomes chipped and irregular, and weight-bearing through the joint becomes uneven.

As a result of uneven distribution of weight, abnormal bony outgrowths start to form around the edges of the joint. These are called 'exostoses' and they never fail to alarm patients when they see them on their X-rays. Then the joints become swollen as synovial fluid pours into the joint space carrying large cartilage-eating cells. These cells are liberated to devour all the accumulated floating fragments of chipped cartilage which have started to clog the joint.

18 An arthritic synovial joint.

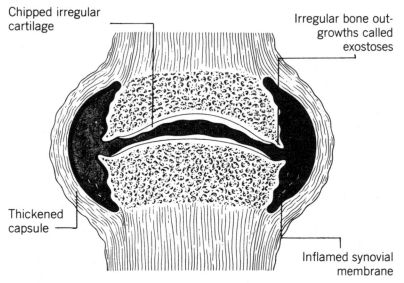

Chipped irregular cartilage

Irregular bone out-growths called exostoses

Thickened capsule

Inflamed synovial membrane

However, when osteo-arthritis becomes painful, the pain does not necessarily come from the bony changes, even those unsightly knobbles of bone. It comes from two separate sources: mechanical irritation and chemical irritation of the tissues of the joint.

Mechanical irritation arises when the soft tissues binding a joint together are stretched. This happens in an acute condition while the joint is swollen and the soft tissues of the joint are stretched by all the fluid trapped in the joint. It also happens in an older, chronic condition when a joint has become tight and will not 'give' with movement. Everyday movement can provoke a stretch on the tight capsule and produce pain. So instead of movement being painless and effortless it becomes painful and laboured.

Chemical irritation is different. Pain in this case comes from the irritating effects of what we call 'inflammatory products'. Inflammation of living tissue happens routinely when that tissue is subjected to trauma or disease. Wherever there is inflammation there are substances produced which by their presence alone irritate nerve endings in living tissue. This registers as pain. This is called chemical irritation and this is how inflammation alone, without the mechanical component, creates pain.

The good news about arthritis is that the condition is partially rectifiable. It is not actually possible to reverse the bony changes, but they were not causing pain anyway. It is possible, however, by simple movement, to pump away unwanted collections of excess fluid in a joint, and this will render the joint less painful. Secondly, movement also softens thickened tissue. This rejuvenates tired old soft tissues that are binding up a joint too tightly. And it is possible for movement to stimulate cartilage regrowth.

It is also thought that this regeneration of cartilage is helped by synovial fluid being pressed or squeezed through the cartilage like water through a sponge as the other bone rolls over it; that the increased movement pushes synovium into parts hitherto not reached, nourishing the cartilage and stimulating regrowth.

At the same time the gristly old soft tissues surrounding the joint, which had been getting thicker and stiffer with lack of activity as time went by, will be stretched and released, then stretched and released again, as the joint undergoes all this healthy new movement. These tissues really have no option but to allow the movement, especially if treatment becomes necessary and a physio like me is pushing that joint around. The surrounding joint tissues gradually slim down and become more elastic and juicy, and then actually quite enjoy moving again. Pain on movement becomes a thing of the past.

Of course you can do this to yourself. In fact I wish you would. However, most people think: 'If it hurts, rest it.' It seems everyone is so terrified of making things worse that they carefully nurse a stiff and painful joint, slowly but surely making the problem into a more serious one.

People have a habit of lying doggo as soon as they feel a pain or hurt. Of course, I do not recommend that you should start flinging yourself about with great gusto as soon as you feel pain, but at least you should keep going — and not grind to a complete halt. Often it is the doctors who rec-ommend rest; it is they who are to be held responsible for the widely used panacea of rest for all physical ailments. Too often they advise that an arm should be put in a sling for three weeks or an ankle needs to go into plaster or a back should go to bed, when gentle progressive movement is what it needs. You must remember that movement is thera-peutic. The freer, smoother, rhythmic action of the joint tends to reduce the swelling and thickening of the soft-tissue structures clothing the joint. The joint becomes younger.

We manual therapists are in the business of making old joints younger. Our professional skill lies in 'bringing a joint on' at the right rate, not in pushing the debilitated joint too hard too soon, before it can take it.

It must be said, though, that in some cases of severe and recent injury to a joint (trauma — the opposite end of the spectrum to the slow, insidious, degenerative changes of osteo-arthritis) that joint may need an initial brief period of rest — between six and twelve hours — but only if it has been very badly wrenched and is still bleeding into the tis-sues. You can tell whether it is still bleeding if the joint becomes increasingly painful. It becomes tenser and tighter as more trapped fluid collects and it will feel hot to the touch. Usually bleeding stops in less than twenty minutes, and thereafter movement should begin. Then the sore joint must be coaxed through the painful unfamiliar movement. Nature only needs a nudge and it will continue the process itself, doing it better and better.

I HAVE RHEUMATOID ARTHRITIS BUT CAN YOU HELP ME?

Rheumatoid arthritis can be an appallingly relentless disease involving permanent pain and disability of most of the joints. In this way it is altogether different from osteo-arthritis which is a much more manageable process, possibly only affecting one joint and easily stopped in the early stages. But there is some good news for the rheumatoid arthritic. It relates to the 'acquired' elements of the joints' affliction. As described previously, osteo-arthritis is caused by damage to the joints, whether by protracted postural strain or by a one-off incident like breaking a leg. In either case, the joint is discommoded and over time the strain tells, hastening its aging process and ultimately its decline.

However, with rheumatoid disease, inflammation itself may be the factor making the joint run badly in the first place. We do not really have the full picture on rheumatoid arthritis but there is increasing evidence that it is a disturbance of the body's immune system, which creates widespread internal inflammation. The result is that the joints hurt. In severe cases, they are hot and even noisy when they move. The patient instinctively learns to adopt any 'antalgic' (pain-relieving) position which will bring some respite from the agony. For instance, he or she would know well the best position in which to sleep: gently on the side and bolstered by pillows, with all the joints — knees, hips, shoulders, elbows and fingers — slightly bent.

Their restricted variety of actions combined with a tendency to remain within the relative safety of their antalgic postures, means that acutely rheumatoid skeletons barely move. Unlike someone suffering from incipient osteo-arthritis, who is trapped by bad habits, the rheumatoid skeleton is trapped by pain. Both syndromes beget pain, but in the case of the rheumatoid arthritic, ever more pain.

This, I believe, is much overlooked in the management of these patients. The pattern of the illness is always that of acute phases fading into chronic or less angry phases. Each successive 'bad phase' leaves the joints more and more bent, the recent acquisitions of deformity super-imposing themselves on the last. A lot of pain comes from these twisted joints. Admittedly, some of it comes from the pure inflammation of the disease itself, but much pain comes from the acquired malfunctionings of the joints, an element which can with vigilant attention, be controlled. As soon as the acute phase is over, the changes have to be redressed.

The important point to stress is that the acquired dysfunction dramatically worsens the pain. Joints that run badly give you pain — even without being rheumatoid.

Each wracking grimace of the joints must be tenderly released before the next real attack, or functional disorder will superimpose itself upon inflammatory disorder and deterioration will be rapid. We must catch the contractures before they become fixed. This means stretching those joints; opening them out. Daily. It will be uncomfortable but well worth the price. Effective management of acute flare-up phases always involves the administration of radical drugs including anti-inflammatories, gold injections or cortisone. You may also have physiotherapy sessions to help straighten the limbs, or better still yoga, if you can manage it (see 'Sport And The Back' Chapter 7).

Rest has always played a prominent role in the short-term management. But of rest and rest alone, I am sceptical. The best approach is joint mobilisation in combination with heavy drug dosages to control the resultant reaction. Rest if you like between stretching sessions. You will need it.

DO I HAVE SCIATICA?

Sciatica is pain in the leg caused by trouble in the back.

At each intervertebral joint level, a pair of spinal nerves which have branched off the spinal cord leave the spine through a small hole between two adjacent vertebrae on either side of the spinal column. The spinal nerves then continue on, outside the spine and into the legs to supply power to the muscles and sensation to the skin. Any structure that gets in the way and irritates the nerve on its way out of the spinal column will cause 'sciatica'.

Sure enough, on their way through these exit canals the spinal nerves pass close by the intervertebral disc on one side and the facet joint on the other. It is unfortunate indeed that a sensitive little nerve must run the gauntlet between two potential aggressors, either of which can readily become swollen and distorted by degenerative change or trauma and inflict themselves upon this fragile strand of nervous tissue.

The whole body is a map of different areas on the skin, the sensation (or feeling) of which is supplied by all the different nerve roots. The exact areas (dermatomes) vary slightly from one person to the next, but it is possible to deduce which nerve root in the spine is being squashed and irritated by finding out exactly where in the leg there is pain or a disturbance of sensation. If the sciatica is very severe, numbness and muscle weakness may also develop. Discs have been blamed as the trouble-makers for years. If you had sciatica, you had a 'disc problem'. 'A disc has slipped and is pinching a nerve.' But how wide off the mark that glib, if persuasive, diagnosis can be. This is just not the way discs behave. Discs never slip anywhere, in or out. They simply bulge and, even if they do bulge, that bulge may be harmless.

Thousands of clinical papers have been written on the subject of the bulging (or slipped) disc — an average of two a week over the past thirty years. We in the medical profession have been brainwashed and as a result have not dared to stray from the old doctrines. Remember that even for medi-

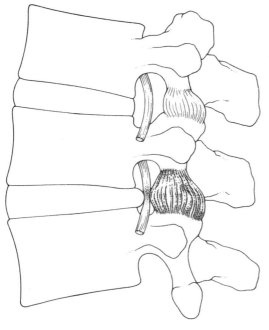

19 Sciatica is brought about by irritation of a spinal nerve.

cal people it is very daunting to witness a fellow-human enduring awful pain. And remember, too, that if one is placed in the position of taking charge there is safety to be had in numbers; safety to be had in all sharing the same professional opinion about a diagnosis. No wonder that change was slow to be realised.

However, gradually the general body of medical opinion is changing. After enjoying an unchallenged reign for fifty-odd years, the dynasty of the disc is dying. Recently, one team of medical researchers came up with the finding that in approximately two-thirds of all operated cases of sciatica the disc was *not* responsible for causing sciatica. These statistics are pretty astounding, especially since they only refer to backs which were serious enough to be actually opened up to allow a look inside.

Most backpain is a simple joint problem, the back's equivalent, you might say, of a twisted ankle. There is too much talk of discs. Discs rarely press on nerves to cause sciatica. It is far more likely that the nerve is subjected to pressure from a swollen and angry facet joint sitting beside the spinal nerve. So often the patient with a backache holds his back. He is telling you where the site of the simple joint dysfunction is and telling you that it will be comforted by the 'laying on of hands'. He often unwittingly rubs it himself to gain relief. When expert thumbs home in on that sore joint, the patient will be surprised to have the painful joint so quickly pinpointed. That characteristic sweet pain; they all say 'That's the spot'! Relief is literally at hand.

But in truth the doctors have been slow to appreciate the worth of manual treatment of backpain. It seems that something as disarmingly 'low-tech' as a simple swollen joint, so easily felt by experienced hands and so readily manipulated free of its swollen and congested state by those hands, was just too uncomplicated for words! It had to be something more high-powered than that.

Another aspect of the disc myth that must be dispelled is that discs suddenly bulge, rupture or pop out. The extremely common claim, made by many a patient, will run loosely as follows: 'Well, I was bending over to pick up the dog and I slipped a disc.' Disc bulges never occur quickly. They take ages.

In their healthy state, discs are extremely robust and inert. They will only start to bulge after they have become weakened and degenerated by years of previous grumbling back trouble. Scientifically controlled experiments where a healthy spine is progressively subjected to increased weight-loading eventually crush the vertebra to a bony rubble while the good old disc remains sitting there happily intact, no bulges. Equally as unlikely in real life is the myth that the discs all sit there like a stack of upside-down saucers just waiting to 'slip out' with one ill-chosen movement. So many people mislead themselves by believing that they have a problem disc that pops in and out on a whim. Discs are extremely strongly attached — indeed, embedded into the bone of the vertebrae between which they sit — so they never slide out from between the bones like a dislodged washer.

While discussing the topic of sciatic pain, we should look at another type of pain which can occur in the leg, in the same distribution as sciatica, but which is 'referred' pain, not sciatica proper. The difference is academic. As a sufferer, you do not much care what is causing that pain in the leg. You just want to get rid of it.

A well-known example of referred pain is a heart attack, and in truth it is a case of the brain misinterpreting where the messages of alarm are coming from. The pain is sometimes felt in the left arm and up the left side of the neck into the jaw — but in fact the trouble is with the heart.

Referred leg pain associated with back trouble is not brought about by direct irritating pressure on the sciatic nerve roots. The mechanism which brings about referred pain is probably as follows.

When a spinal facet joint is inflamed and painful because it is in trouble, its own nerve supply picks up the messages of pain. This is felt as pain in the back and is the most common cause of backache.

However, it is possible that other structures sharing the same nerve supply as that inflamed joint will also feel pain. It could be the sensation to the skin of the lower leg or that of the thin filmy tissue covering the bones of the lower leg, but either way you have a nagging vague pain in the buttock, hip or leg quite far distant from the low back. However, it is the problem in the back which is the source of the trouble and the pain in the leg is the effect.

It is thought that the patient perceives the leg to be painful because, although the skin of that part of the leg shares its nerve supply with the problem level in the back, the skin has a much 'richer' nerve supply than the joint in the back, and the brain, in error, assumes the leg to be the part of the body that needs be taken care of. In the jargon of the academics, referred pain is experienced in that part of the body 'with the greatest receptor density'.

It would be fair to say that all of us in the profession are pretty vague about pain, particularly referred pain. There is a lot we do not understand, especially phenomena such as referred tenderness. How on earth does that happen?

The other state of affairs which can complicate an already complicated picture is that after a lengthy period of time spent suffering referred pain, eventually the structures underlying the painful area, far removed from the source of the trouble, will themselves start to function badly and become painful. This happens because we unwittingly attempt to spare the part too much activity. We reduce our demands on the underlying joint, or use it in an awkward way, which ultimately causes it to start functioning badly, with pain as the result.

So it is not uncommon for somebody to come to me and say: 'I've got this pain in my hip' or 'My knee feels weak'. I will always check the hip or knee, which may indeed show signs of minimal dysfunction, possibly responsible for some of the pain, but invariably the real problem is up in the back.

Referred pain is a curious phenomenon, but it is distinguishable from sciatic pain, firstly, because it will be a more vague pain with less well-defined borders and, secondly, the sciatic nerve will not be sensitive to stretch. Inflamed nervous tissue is very sensitive to being stretched. But if it is referred leg pain and not pure 'sciatica' the nerve itself will not be irritable.

If it is pure sciatica, the nerve itself is inflamed and irritable and it will be more than usually sensitive to stretch. The way to stretch the nerve to find out is to allow the leg to be raised off the bed straight up to as close to ninety degrees as possible. With severe irritability, the leg barely gets two inches off the bed before there is a severe increase of the leg pain. Stretching the nerve even to that slight degree aggravates it.

With referred leg pain, this classical 'straight leg raise' will be painless. The nerve itself is not involved directly in the inflammatory process and is therefore not sensitive.

IS IT MY SACRO-ILIAC JOINT?

Most probably not.

There was a time when the twisted sacro-iliac or the

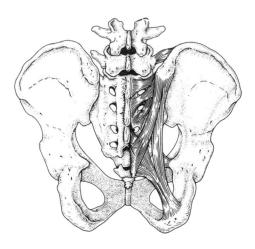

20 *The sacro-iliac joints join the base of the spine to the pelvis. They are bound together by a tenacious criss-crossing lattice of ligament.*

twisted pelvis was definitely in vogue. Everybody had one. Every vague pain from the small toe to the naval was attributed to bad goings-on in this joint. However, with better techniques for diagnosis that have been developed in recent years, we now see things a little differently.

If anything is going to go wrong with the low lumbar area, it is far more likely to be the spine than either sacro-iliac joint. Even with all that repetitive, poorly controlled bending we do all the time — bad bending localised to the bottom two hinges of the spine — the sacro-iliac joints get by largely unstressed. Why should they complain? The back does all the work. The two sacro-iliac joints bind the pelvis to the sacrum at the base of the spine where the two dimples are to be seen at the bottom of the back. They are fantastically strong joints, bound front and back with powerful inelastic ligaments which allow only the smallest degree of movement of the pelvis, rather like the unwilling 'give' of dense plastic. It is far more difficult to strain these two joints, therefore, than it is to strain the spine, that tall willowy structure rising out of the pelvis so vulnerable to every kind of jolt and bang.

In medicine there is a saying: 'Common things are common.' In this instance, it is far more common for a fragile little lumbar spinal joint to be hurt in an accidental jolt than one of the big sacro-iliac joints set so secure and bound-up, deep within the pelvis. However, there are times when a sacro-iliac joint can get strained. It is, as we have seen, hardly likely to happen incidentally. Rather, the accident that causes this injury must be a fairly dramatic one; a sitting-down fall on to the bottom, especially if one buttock hits the ground first, or perhaps a Rugby scrum collapsing on the man underneath (in this case the player was already bent forward, so his spine, being fully curled, was relatively stable, and therefore the sacro-iliac joint was the structure to get strained).

Another way of straining a sacro-iliac joint comes about when one leg is shorter than the other by more than a centimetre or so (see 'What is the Short Leg Syndrome', later in the chapter). This is a more subtle type of strain which comes on slowly over years. The joint complains when one hip is higher than the other because there is unequal sharing of the body's weight.

Strain is brought about by a twisting action of either side of the pelvis either forwards and down or upwards and back around the sacrum in the middle, which does not move.

The treatment of a strained sacro-iliac joint is just the same as treating any other joint. The legacy of that strain is stiffness. The joint will be loath to move in one or more directions. To treat the joint and get rid of the pain is to find which direction it does not want to go in — and then persuade it to do so! Find the stiffness and unstiffen it.

The osteopaths like to talk about displacement forwards or backwards, and how it is necessary to correct this misalignment — usually with hefty manipulations to force it around into a more pleasing anatomical position. I feel this is the 'ideal' rather than the 'real' approach. We manual therapists tackle the problem differently. Our approach is to correct the 'movement blockage' and let it find its own position in its own time — which it will do if it is not manhandled too much.

Our technique is generally to loosen the half-pelvis so that it is freer to move in any way it chooses. As a natural follow-on from this, any displacement will realign itself spontaneously if it wants to, the negative and positive contours on the two opposing joint surfaces getting together and notching in as readily as they possibly can.

It is the gentle rejuvenation of the tissues binding the joint, changing them from dry and tight to supple and elastic, which transforms a joint from a painful to a painless one. The position of the bones is unimportant. It is simply the stiffness which causes the pain, and any misalignment persists because that stiffness is not allowing it to return to its natural 'untwisted' position.

The manual techniques we use must be fairly hefty because the joint is so strong and immobile, even in its healthy state. The easiest way for me to do it is to lie the patient face down and then get my knee on to the prominent ledge of bone beside the dimple of the painful side. I then kneel up on it and sort of trample the joint. I can feel it 'giving' under me as it starts to move more and more freely. It does not hurt at all except for that typical 'sweet pain' which comes about when the problem is put under pressure and which is such a relief for you, the patient, to feel.

There is another type of sacro-iliac trouble associated with pregnancy, which is not purely the result of physical strains of the joint. It comes about not because the sacro-iliac joints are too stiff but because they are too loose.

During the later stages of pregnancy a hormone is liberated which acts on the ligaments of the pelvis to soften them. This is to allow the pelvis to separate slightly during labour so that the baby can pass through more freely during deliv-

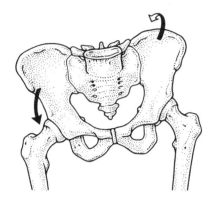

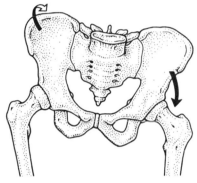

21 Twisting strains of either side of the pelvis around a central fixed sacrum.

ery. This loose pelvis can be painful, and also by being loose it is vulnerable to injury thereafter.

After my second baby, as a matter of interest, I had just this problem. Every time I stood on one leg to put on my tights, there was a definite clonk and shuffle as one side of my pelvis slid upwards in relation to the other — but, then, I had been pushing and tugging a string of patients about until the evening before my labour. . . .

Such an unstable, loose sacro-iliac joint gradually tightens up again in time. Mine did. It's barely painful in the meantime, and I'm back on top again.

Sometimes — we do not know why — this sloppy state continues and is a real problem to deal with. The best thing to be done is to bind the pelvis together with a sacro-iliac brace, a four-inch-wide belt worn tightly around the hips below the stomach to try to pull the pelvis together artificially.

HAVE I AN EXTRA VERTEBRA?

The human spine sits atop the table-like upper surface of the sacrum which is a solid mass of bone making up the back wall of the pelvis. The surface of the table tilts downward quite dramatically at the front, which means that, having originated on the sacrum, the spine must arch backwards as it rises out of the pelvis to bring itself back over the centre of gravity. The greater the forward tip of the sacrum, therefore, the more the spine will have to double back, creating a greater lumbar hollow. Some individuals have a sacral angle which is almost flat, with little resultant lumbar lordosis, whereas others have a sacral angle approaching 90 degrees. In this latter instance it can be seen how properties of the sacrum may influence the workings of the spine above. In the case of too much sacral tip, the problems are related to shearing forces of the spine as it tends to slip forward off the sacral base.

There is another set of anomalies of the sacrum which have a direct influence on the activity of the spine above.

In earlier evolutionary forms of the humanoid skeleton, it is believed that the sacrum was a primitive version of a tail, in which the sacral vertebral segments moved in concert with the rest of the spine. In modern man, however, the sacrum is solid. It is a rigid block of five fused vertebrae on which the upright spine sits.

There are two congenital anomalies of the block-like sacrum which can also influence the workings of the spine above. 'Lumbarisation' is where the uppermost segment of the sacrum, instead of being fused, is loose and participates along with the neighbouring lumbar segments in spinal activity. The first sacral segment is said to be 'lumbarised'. Anatomists and clinicians have taken to referring to this ad-

22 The difference between a great sacral angle and almost no sacral angle.

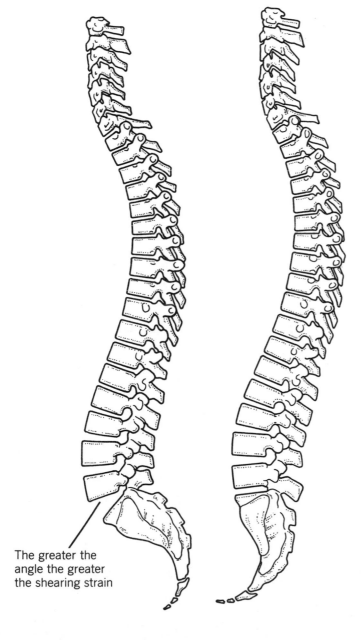

The greater the angle the greater the shearing strain

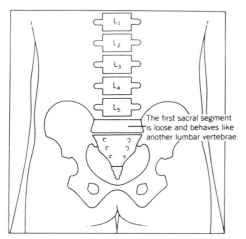

The first sacral segment is loose and behaves like another lumbar vertebrae.

23.1 Lumbarisation

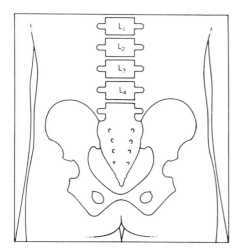

23.2 Sacralisation

ditional mobile lumbar segment as an extra vertebra, something I feel which has led to much confusion. There is no extra vertebra jammed into the length of the spine, but simply one extra mobile vertebra and one less fused or fixed vertebra.

The other congenital anomaly is where the bottom lumbar segment (L5), is fused to the sacrum, so there is one less mobile vertebra in the spine and an extra fused one. As such it has more in common with its sacral neighbours than its lumbar brethren so it is said to be 'sacralised'.

It has always been assumed that such findings are clinically unimportant but I can't agree. Generally speaking, I believe they both cause trouble because of the incomplete nature of the phenomena. With lumbarisation, it is rare for this additional joint to be completely free and with sacralisation, it is rare for this joint to be absolutely fused. The pure extreme of both anomalies is not commonly found. Usually, the problem joint is neither here nor there but in a no man's land, neither completely loose nor completely fixed. There is a certain safety to be had in a joint being completely fused, which helps to explain the penchant of orthopaedic surgeons (though less common these days) for fusing problem joints. The rationale had always been, drastic as it was, that if a joint hurt to move, better stop it moving. That this inevitably led to other problems in the nearby mobile joints, which were sometimes as unwelcome as the original complaint, is another matter; the case for fusion can be clearly seen. However, if the fusions did not work then everybody was in a quandary. Indeed, surgical fusions that do not quite 'take' have always been the bane of the back surgeon's life.

Exactly the same is true of Nature's fusions. Those that are not quite solid are a problem. Again, to use the analogy of another joint, if you jump off a wall onto a slightly stiff ankle, you run the risk of hurting it by landing heavily upon it. The joint is simply not loose enough to roll with the action and absorb the shock. It will be badly jarred and it will swell and be painful. On the other hand, if the joint is as good as new, it will be no problem at all to land on. It is free enough of movement to take the shock and keep going. Conversely if it were fused rock-solid, though the landing might judder your frame, the joint would not suffer.

In short, it is better for a joint to be one way or the other, either freely mobile or rock solid, if it is to deflect trauma. Half-way between the two is a highly vulnerable state of affairs. Invariably with sacralised fifth lumbar segments, the fusion is not quite solid; if it were it would remain un-enticed by nearby movement. As it is, I believe such joints contribute to a small degree in the overall movement. And like any other joint which is lacking in mobility, the movement which it does have is not good enough. As described at length elsewhere in this book, the same scenario evolves where a poorly functioning joint sets itself up as an easy target for further damage. Strain heaps itself upon old damage and creates new damage and more strain. The joint's health and consequently its function, deteriorates. Pain is the result.

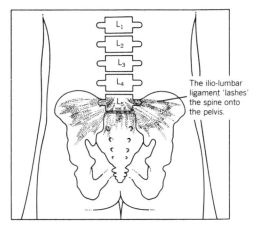

24 *The ilio-lumbar ligament.*

The ilio-lumbar ligament 'lashes' the spine onto the pelvis.

I find that exactly the converse is true of spines which demonstrate lumbarisation of the first sacral segment. Admittedly, that extra joint between the first and second sacral segment is said to be free, but in truth, it is not free enough. Again the spine is caught in no man's land, attempting to effortlessly incorporate this additional joint in its everyday function. But invariably this 'ring-in' joint is not up to the task. Though it is said to be mobile it is not quite loose enough and it is vulnerable. Normal movement tweaks it, because the effort is too much to cope with. Like the one which is meant to be fused, it also gets hurt. My solution is to get both types, the semi-fused and the semi-free, moving. Attempting to get movement into a radiologically fixed joint always strikes my fellow medical practitioners as bizarre, but treatment is usually short-term and usually rewarding for the patient. All the usual self-mobilisation exercises described in this book can be put into action. Sacralisation also has another far-reaching effect, one not associated with joint mobility. This one relates to the altered centre of gravity of the spine. It comes about because the lowest mobile segment is much higher, making the base of the spine less secure. Normally the spine originates deep within the pelvis and it is safe down there, anchored by a three dimensional spread of ligamentous stays. The ligaments fan out in a dense semi-circle from the fifth lumbar vertebra to the pelvis, and lash the spine onto the sacral table. It is a masterpiece of design.

The most mobile joint in the spine in terms of bending and straightening is that between L4 and L5. But L4 derives security for its flamboyant activity by L5 in turn acting as a sturdy mobile base. This partly explains why the lowest lumbar vertebra, L5, displays such relative paucity of freedom. But it also explains why, when L5 has no movement because it has become fused, the next level up, L4, is

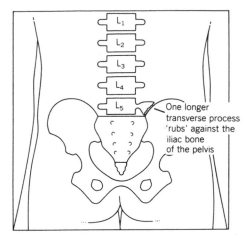

25.1 Unilateral transverse sacralisation

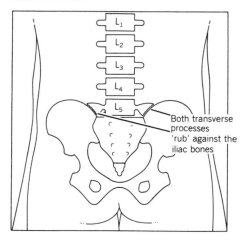

25.2 Bilateral transverse sacralisation

vulnerable when taking over the role. Though L4 readily compensates for inaction at L5, it does so deprived of the substantial ligamentous shoring afforded L5. In taking on the brunt of the movement with L5 out of action, L4 is ill-equipped for the task. The flimsy joint between L4 and L5 is exposed to excessive strain. It becomes over-used and eventually painful, a problem endemic to the sacralised L5.

Treatment of these disorders entails not only mobilisation of the fused fifth lumbar segment, but muscle strengthening of the union between the fourth and fifth lumbar vertebrae, not unlike the techniques used to shore up developmental hyper-mobility as a result of surgical fusion (see 'Do I Need an Operation?' Chapter 4).

In each case, overuse creates an incipient sloppiness of the vertebral link. This cannot be allowed to continue, otherwise surgical fusion will be necessary, progressively higher up the spine. Intrinsic spinal-strengthening exercise is essential to pre-empt this. Straightening the spine in a unfurling fashion from the fully curled position, will bind together the overused link above the fusion (see diagrams 53.1 to 53.3, Chapter 6). As an exercise it must be done without fail at least three or four times a week, ideally after having performed the rolling exercises on the floor as described at the end of Chapter 6 to limber the spine beforehand. Before moving on from this subject of sacralisation, there is yet another version of the condition which brings with it another set of problems. Every vertebra has several projections or lateral struts of bone which extend out from the central body. There are the two transverse processes on either side, and a single spinous process at the back. (You can see these as knobs which protrude through the skin all the way down the back). Sometimes the transverse processes of the fifth lumbar vertebra are so long that they impinge on the two iliac bones (and sometimes the sacrum as well) either side of the spine. In this way too the fifth lumbar vertebra is said to be sacralised. In this case however, the central junction between the body of L5 and the sacrum is usually fully or at least partly operative. The main obstruction to free mobility of the bottom lumbar segment is created by the transverse process grinding against the ilia with every movement. Nature copes with the bone-to-bone rub with its usual ingenuity; a false joint comes into being to lubricate the junction. Even so, streamlined movement is seriously hampered.

An even greater impediment to graceful movement occurs when only one transverse process is longer than usual and impinges on the ilium while the other swings free. Here again, the abnormal union is either fused solid or, if there is some movement, a false joint develops. Either way, lumbar mobility is severely disturbed by this unilateral jamming. Every movement of the lumbar spine is accompanied by a slewing-around effect as the spine tries to move away from the pelvis but cannot because it is unilaterally tethered. Again, the method of treatment is to attempt to release the binding nature of the abnormal joint by manually mobilising it to get more movement. This type of sacralisation is surprisingly easy to feel. As I probe around the side of the flat sacral mass, the presence of the false junction is obvious by its bony quality, almost as if it is just under the skin. If the condition were normal, there would be nothing there to feel.

Investigating thumbs have no difficulty at all in sensing the degree of movement it harbours. When it comes to getting it un-jammed however, the thumbs alone are usually not strong enough. This is where the elbow comes in! I use the point of the elbow with the arm fully bent, exerting pressure down the shaft of my upper arm. I direct the push laterally against the ledge of the ilium so as to prise the pelvis off the spine. It hurts but it works.

WHAT IS THE SHORT LEG SYNDROME?

In a preceding section, 'Is it my Sacro-Iliac Joint?', the shortness of one leg was nominated as a possible cause of chronic though mild sacro-iliac disorders. However, a discrepancy in leg length can lead to other manifestations of pain in the lower back which may be termed: 'The Short Leg Syndrome'. Over a period of years, someone with legs of slightly differing length unconsciously evens up the tilt of the pelvis by tending to stand with the longer leg slightly bent at the hip and the knee, often placing the foot of the longer leg slightly ahead of the other on the floor. This gradually causes changes in the mobility of the hip of the longer leg, which eventually affects the functioning of the spine as a whole. Signs of adaptive shortening of the soft tissue and muscles running across the front of that hip become apparent, as it loses the ability to straighten out. This process of 'flexion contracture', as it is called, takes place so insidiously that it can only be detected by clinical assessment and not even the sufferer is aware of its happening.

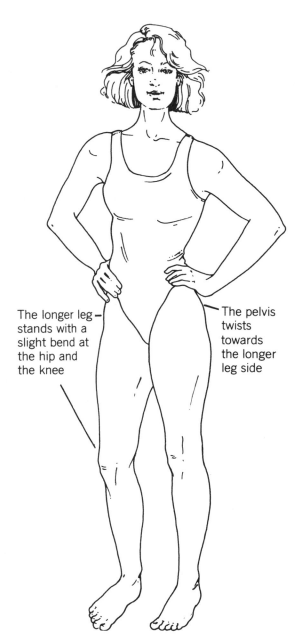

The longer leg stands with a slight bend at the hip and the knee

The pelvis twists towards the longer leg side

26 The short leg syndrome.

However, inequality of hip freedom especially in a backward direction can have serious consequences for a spine, most markedly during walking. When one goes to take a step forward on the short leg, it must of necessity be of reduced length as the hip of the longer leg does not have sufficient 'give' to angle back to the desired degree. The pelvis must twist towards the longer leg to compensate partly for the lack of freedom of that hip. This pelvic rotation creates a relative internal rotation of the hip of the longer leg together with a 'pronation' or forcing downwards of the front of the foot.

Also, the low back must constantly adapt to the downward slope of the pelvis towards the side of the shorter leg. The spine also must cope with the greater freedom of one hip over the other. During walking, the spine is forced to twist one way to compensate for the lack of contribution from the hip. With each step on the short leg, the spine must twist to the side of the long leg, to make up for the lack of 'give' from that hip. This puts a constant strain on the machinery of the lower back.

Because of their anatomical alignment, the facet joints of the lumbar spine allow very little twisting mobility. On the other hand, the alignment of the facets in the thoracic spine is in a plane which encourages one vertebra to swivel on another. Furthermore, the change in facet alignment in the lumbar spine to that in the thoracic spine is quite abrupt. As the demand for twist comes up from the hips, the paucity of twist of the lumbar spine means that all the lumbar vertebrae move as a rigid block, until the movement reaches the facets in the thoracic spine with their different alignment. At this point (at high waist level) massive de-rotation takes place. With every step on the shorter leg the thoraco-lumbar junction collects an excessive twist, with the result that 'over-use' strain develops here.

The first step in dealing with this syndrome is to correct the leg length discrepancy. A cork or rubber insole is best, though this is only suitable for flatter shoes. But it obviates the need for building up the heel of the shoe by a bootmaker. Women's shoes usually do need to have the heel built up, but not the sole unless the discrepancy is great. Under-correction is usually desirable. Scrupuiously accurate measurement to the nearest millimetre is not necessary. The skeleton has learnt to adapt over the years and over-zealous correction may be too great a shock to the system. One simply attempts to minimise the difference.

The next step is to assess the relative freedom of both the

hips, particularly in the direction of extension (the backward movement). This is best done by lying flat on your back on a bed, firstly close to the right-hand edge so that the right leg is unsupported and hangs over the side (see diagram 45, Chapter 6). Hold the left leg around the knee and pull it as high up to the chest as possible. This will cause the right leg to move upwards correspondingly. The tighter the hip, the higher this leg will lift off the floor, with a greater sensation of 'pulling' across the front of the hip and upper thigh. If there is no tightness present, the leg will not lift off the floor. Some hips are so tight that they passively levitate to well above the horizontal. To compare this with the left leg, move across to the other side of the bed and repeat the action by hugging the right leg to the chest. Differences of freedom are immediately apparent, the short leg usually being much looser than the long.

This difference in freedom has to be redressed before the back problem can be resolved. The best stretch is the modified yoga lunge. If the left leg is longer, it will be this hip which is tighter. Take up a stride position with the left foot across at right angles and the right foot, about a metre directly in front of it, facing straight ahead. Lunge down on the right knee so that it bends to a 90 degree angle. With the left hip thus opened, you will feel a good stretch, which encourages extension and external rotation of the longer leg. It should be repeated three or four times daily. Take great care not to allow your back to form a deep hollow, a trick movement to spare the hip. Keep your pelvis rotated well back. Check the comparative freedom of movement by applying the same stretch to the other hip at least once each session.

Lastly, the spine needs to be assessed again for its mobility. It usually twists one way more happily than it does the other, the result of a twisted walking pattern over a long period. Thumbs can easily detect resistance to the swing in the individual vertebrae. They will also detect a lack of resistance from the opposite direction, as if the movement is 'empty' or unobstructed. Full bilateral rotation must be restored.

You can partly do this yourself. The best rotation exercise is to lie on the floor with your knees bent, arms spread out. When twisting the knees to the right, cross your right knee over the left at the knee and let both roll towards the floor. This will open out the left hand side of the spine and also exert traction on the spine. Repeat the action to the left with

27 The yoga lunge.

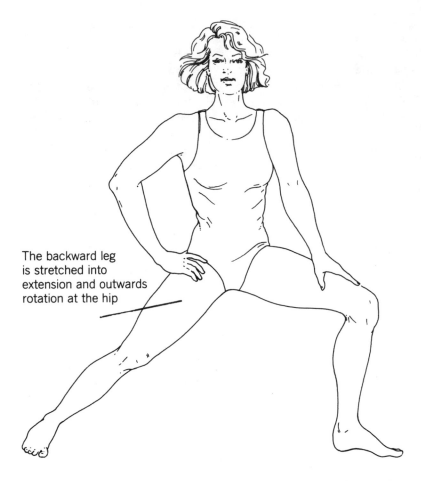

The backward leg is stretched into extension and outwards rotation at the hip

the left knee cocked over. Roll several times in the 'tight' direction for every single roll in the looser direction.

The tightness of hip on the side of the longer leg also needs to be corrected. Tightness here nods the pelvis forward so that the lower back forms a deep hollow (see diagram 35, Chapter 6), something which hampers the self-stacking arrangement of the spine and creates shear.

But there is another important reason why hip flexor tightness should be checked. Research has shown that over-activity of the powerful hip flexor group causes reciprocal weakness of the stomach muscles; that group so vital to the support of the spine. The fact that tight hip flexors are the chief inhibitors of a strong tummy is a powerful incentive to ensure that the hips get fixed. It is even more important therefore, to read the section on sit-ups (see 'What Exercises Should I Do?', Chapter 6) since doing them badly will only add to your problems. No other exercise has the capacity to help you or to hinder you, depending on whether you do it well. Done well, sit-ups can cure a back problem. Done badly, they can cause one. So, in order to keep our backs in shape, we have to keep our stomachs in shape and in order to keep our stomachs in shape we have to keep our hips in shape. As simple as that.

WHAT IS SPINAL SCOLIOSIS?

The longer I spend in problem back management, the more I find myself interested in the condition called scoliosis. It seems to get so overlooked! Mild cases are often dismissed as malingering. Quasimodo, the Hunchback of Notre Dame had scoliosis, though to a grotesque degree not often seen today. Scoliosis is curvature of the spine. From behind, instead of being straight it displays 'S'-shaped curve which may be shockingly marked or barely noticeable. In Quasimodo's case, his hideous hump, so cunningly re-created by the movie make-up artists, was his rib cage, twisted around and thrust up like a fin.

With the screening of school children, together with better diet and heightened medical awareness, the disorder rarely deteriorates to the same degree. However, mild to moderate cases of scoliosis are extremely common. Studies have shown that many people have a slight curve concave to the right in the mid-thoracic area, probably because of the predominance of right-handedness and also the position of the aorta in the chest cavity. It is the mild cases which are the most daunting, because it is not unusual for adolescent boys and girls to complain of pain everywhere: headaches, pain in the neck, under the shoulder blades, in the lower back and sometimes down the legs. It is common to see the families and their doctors at their wits end. Scolioses usually manifest themselves during adolescence during sudden growth spurts. Whatever the other factors, it seems that the rapid bone growth compared to the comparatively slower soft tissues growth, means that the spine becomes caught in a web of its own soft tissues as it shoots skyward. What starts as a transient correctable hint of a bend, quickly becomes fixed. Month by month, the deformity becomes more pronounced and the children are powerless. With the mild ones, the most effective remedy is vigorous sporting activity. Some formal side-bending also helps, to 'undo' the bend. Yoga is excellent. Countless theories have been put forward to explain scoliosis, though attention has always focused on the severe cases. Growing opinion claims that the mild cases are the result of sub-clinical cases of cerebral palsy with its inequality of muscle tone on either side of the body. Such 'spastic'

28 Spinal scoliosis

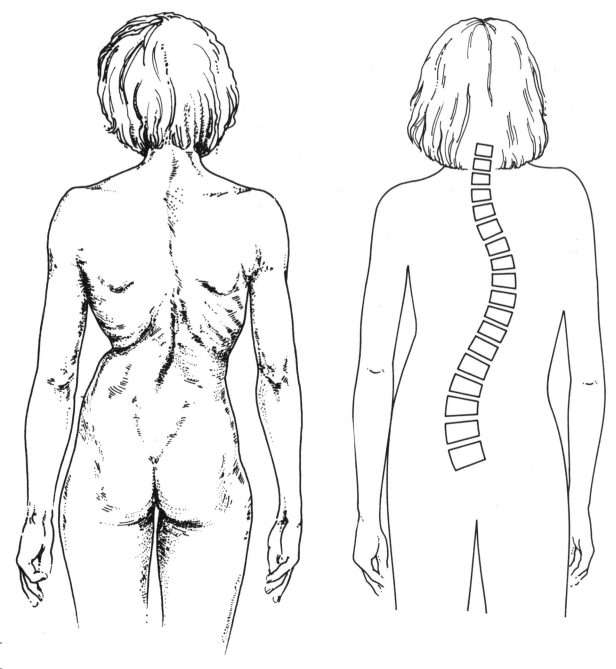

conditions in children are often hard to detect. The child might be slightly clumsier than its peers, slightly behind in its 'motor milestones' — the appropriate level of physical ability for its age — and it is often this that worries the parents more than the spinal changes. Whatever the cause, scoliosis is often debilitating. Adolescents bring on its symptoms with a rush with their fast growing, their carrying of heavy school bags and their sitting studying for long hours. But depending on the severity of the curve and the amount of physical activity in one's youth, the strain of the curve may not make itself felt until later life when the elasticity of our tissues naturally starts to fade.

Normal vertebrae resemble house bricks. They have flat top and bottom surfaces with hard edges to maintain dynamic stability as the column sits upon itself and moves. The spine achieves equilibrium by self-stacking, with each vertebra exactly centred above the one below, to create perfect harmony. Admittedly muscle power is required once it shifts out of an upright position but even so, the mechanics of the spine are a remarkably efficient, stable arrangement. But if the stacking arrangement of the spine is off-centre, it never achieves complete dynamic equilibrium. As it falls out of alignment, it slews around upon itself and bends.

In scoliosis, a distinction is made between primary and secondary curves of the spine, with the secondary curve developing to balance the primary below. It is a compensatory factor to keep the centre of gravity over the pelvis and at the top of the column, to keep the eyes level.

Over time this disturbed balance of the spine, first one way and then the other, leads to a plethora of subtle strains. As the spine tries to resist the bending forces, pain is created by several simultaneous factors — the disequilibrium of muscle power on both sides of the column, the wedge shape of the vertebrae tending to slide sideways off one another, the strain suffered by the restraining ligaments, the jamming of the vertebral hinges on the inside of the curve and in the thoracic area, the skew-whiff bucket handle action of the ribs attempting to key in to the bucking and rolling sides of the thoracic spine. This may explain why moderate to severe cases of scoliosis deteriorate so rapidly.

The surgical correction of such deteriorating curves usually involves the principles of distraction of the spine, as well as shifting the convex hump sideways or inwards. In my opinion, too little use is made of pre-operative manual mobilisation of the scoliotic spine to optimise the post-operative result. However, with mild scoliotics, the combination of manual mobilisation and general stretching exercises to 'prise open' and straighten the spinal hoops brings the best results, both in diminishing pain and retarding further angulation.

Again, in cases of mild and hitherto undiagnosed scolioses, there is a lot to be said for unilateral muscle strengthening exercises on the weakened side of the spine. Any all-round activity like cycling or swimming which makes allowance for a latent weakness of a leg or arm or one side of the trunk will also be of benefit. With manual treatment, there is always a recurring pattern in the location of the problem sites. Gravity causes the half-hoops to bend or squash further so that the joints at the apices of each curve are pinched in the bend of the hoop. On manual examination it is easy to feel these jammed links. Because of the twist in a scoliotic spine, the individual vertebrae will always be semi-locked in a degree of fixed rotation. In clinical practice we find that 'transverse pressures' work well to undo this. These are pressures with the thumbs, sideways against the small knobs of the back. They restore some of the lost rotation, causing an immediate reduction in pain. Pressures to the ribs where they lock in to the sides of the twisted spine, also help. Again, as an overall approach, yoga is invaluable (see section on Yoga, Chapter 7).

WHAT IS VERTEBRAL STENOSIS?

Stenosis is a cramped cord in the spinal canal. It is described in Chapter 4 (see 'Do I Need an Operation?') as a complication of surgical intervention. But stenosis can also be congenitally acquired — you are born with it — or it can be acquired by degenerative changes, when the internal spinal canal steadily silts up with bone and tissue. Whatever the cause, the result is that the spinal cord and the spinal nerves hanging down inside the canal are subjected to a very tight fit. The cramped conditions reduce the margin in which the highly sensitive neural matter can swing around and this leads to trouble.

You do not notice anything amiss while you are inactive but it's a different story as soon as you try and walk up a hill. Normally, during the act of walking, the demand for action invokes an immediate response in the nerves which stimulate the muscles of the legs. The nerves within the canal engorge themselves with blood in order to carry out their function. But if conditions in the spinal canal are too cramped to permit the nerves to swell as they should, the nerves themselves suffer blood starvation, which gives rise to diffuse pains in one or both legs. The pain is only ever evident while walking, be it on the flat, up a slope or up steps. It can be distinguished from pain associated with vascular disease, with which it is often confused, because the pain will intensify over increasingly short distances after you have been forced to rest to relieve it. In severe cases it may be necessary to squat to gain relief, since this broadens the internal dimensions of the canal and allows more blood to get through to the nerves.

Many people have a narrower than usual spinal canal but do not experience stenosis symptoms until some other development further reduces its dimensions. In such cases these space-occupying lesions — most commonly disc bulges or arthritic changes — make a tight fit even tighter.

With degenerative arthritis, there is a proliferation of extra bone and lumpy soft tissues. These deposit themselves everywhere; in and around all the joints and hinges of the spine and as a lumpy internal lining of the spinal canal.

The facet joint is perhaps the junction most readily affected by this process. Stenosis here accounts for the picture of pain in one leg only and is the result of the silting up of a lateral exit canal (the intervertebral foramen). Gross thickening of the facet joint, which forms part of the border of the exit canal creates a calcified stricture around the spinal nerve root as it is on its way out. It is significant to note here that the degeneration of the facet joint often appears to have been a relatively unobtrusive process without much backache. It is often only years later that they complain of the characteristic leg pain. In these cases, the back degeneration was 'cold' rather than 'hot'. Although there may have been 'a bit of a grumbling back over the years' it will generally not have caused the patient anything like the bother of the more recent leg pain. There can be an added complication. If the fuzzing up of the neural canal is accompanied by a degree of spondylolisthesis or forward slip of one vertebra off its neighbour below, the symptoms of vertebral stenosis will be even more marked. The presence of spondylolisthesis creates a step in the inner tube of the spinal canal which produces a collar of constriction on the cord. In slipping out of place the vertebra also makes a bony notch in the diam-

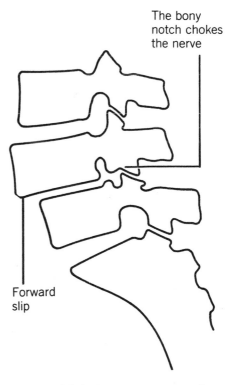

The bony notch chokes the nerve

Forward slip

29 Spondylolisthesis can create a bony notch and occlude the foramen.

eter of the intervertebral foramen which partially occludes the hole through which the spinal nerve has to pass. Both anomalies can give rise to symptoms of stenosis. Furthermore, with spondylolisthesis, the ever-present possibility of increasing shear-slippage of the upper vertebra, results in increased wear and tear, which accelerates the other process. Arthritis on the rampage! The central canal and/or the intervertebral foramen are occluded even more.

Deterioration is insidious and often the final straw is the most trivial of incidents — a rick getting out of the car or tripping over in the garden — and the neural canals become even more fugged-up by local inflammation and swelling.

It is cases like these which support my view on the mixed value of X-rays. They are the ones which almost defy radiologists' powers of description because the pictures look so bad. Yet invariably these are the people who barely knew they had a problem before the causative incident took place. This bodes well though for their prognosis, despite the appalling X-rays. And with appropriate treatment it is not long before their ravaged backs are working as well and painlessly as they ever did.

As with all problem back cases, the critical factor is the degree of internal inflamed engorgement and whether with my hands, I can cause this to subside gently without adding to the general hubbub. Manual therapy works well, especially if it is matched with abdominal muscle strengthening. But even if we cannot shrink the soft-tissue build-up around the nerve root and the back does go to surgery, the post-operative result is much enhanced by pre-operative manual techniques to minimise the congestion and maximise tummy support.

WHAT WILL X-RAYS DO?

X-rays are, without doubt, the most boring aspect of my field of medicine — mainly because everybody is so obsessive about them. They are important to exclude the presence of fractures, rheumatoid arthritis and tumours, but would be about it.

X-rays take 'still' pictures of bones, but bones are not a common cause of pain. It is the *joints*, those junctions of bone, held together by soft tissues, which give the trouble. It is like taking a photograph of a hinge in a door. You cannot tell from the picture whether the hinge works or not. Of course, if there are lumps of rust hanging off it you might fairly safely assume that the running won't be too smooth — but, then, it might be.

There are thousands of instances where there is dreadful backpain but nothing shows up on X-ray, just as there are those where the X-rays are awful but there has never been a day of pain. X-rays can and do pinpoint sites of trouble by showing a joint to be moth-eaten and more irregular in outline than the next; but, as I have said, the one that looks the worst may not be the one which is currently causing the trouble.

However, it would seem that the presence of a problem joint on X-ray may not be entirely divorced from the fact that one does feel pain elsewhere. It would seem that the obvious-looking X-ray changes of gnarled and knobbly joints are rather like the white ashes left after a fierce glowing fire. But the fire has long gone out of that particular joint, the inflammation has died and the ashes are cold. The joint has gone through its agonies some time long ago and is now quiescent. But, as always, the legacy of former inflammation is severe dysfunction of the joint. This in turn will throw excessive strain on to the nearest joint or the next but one. Although the strain of this segment might not be obvious on X-ray, it is actually responsible for causing a lot of discomfort. This phenomenon also accounts for the criss-cross siting of trouble back and forth across to either side of the spine, up and down the entire length of the spine. As a lack of mobility of a single facet on one side makes its effects felt, it translates strain diagonally across to the other side of the spine, criss-crossing the spine back and forth, as it goes up. This is more common in the neck than in the low back and accounts for the often confusing picture of the 'pain everywhere' syndrome.

When this happens, the X-rays might show the joint on the right to be in a deteriorated state, but it is the poor joint a couple of levels up on the other side which is taking all the strain as a result of the one below not working properly. Although there may be pain, the signs of strain may be too early to show up on X-ray: signs of bony change do not start to show up till long after functional performance goes awry. X-rays do not tell us a thing about paucity of function, and that, after all, is the reason for pain. 'Stiffness' does not show up in pictures.

Furthermore, soft-tissue structures are not what is called

'radio-opaque', so regardless of their state of health, they cannot be seen on X-ray, and therefore cannot be shown as troublesome. This includes the discs, which everybody gets so excited about! Bulges cannot be seen. Remember that. The only thing we can deduce about the disc on an X-ray plate is that its height may be diminished, but we certainly cannot see if it is bulging and pressing on or pinching a nerve.

It would be an enormous help if there was such a tool as an X-ray video in use, to see joint performance in action. It would then be a simple job to diagnose, as it moves, which part of the spine is not joining in properly. But as it stands at the moment in practice the only fail-safe way is actually to *feel* the spine as it moves and, while so doing, ask the patient whether each individual joint is painful as each is singled out. If the surgeons are considering an operation, they will do a myelogram or a radiculogram beforehand. This involves injecting a radio-opaque dye into the internal canal space, waiting until it trickles around all the discs and nerve roots, and then X-raying the result. If there is an abnormal bulging contour of the disc which could conceivably be causing pressure damage, they would feel justified in removing the disc. But, apart from that, X-rays are not much use at all. My clinic is piled high with people's abandoned X-rays, so obviously they are as bored with them as I am.

4

A CHOICE OF TREATMENTS

Before I get on to talking about my favourite subject, manual mobilisation, with particular reference to its value in treating the spine, I want to give you a brief survey of all the other treatment choices available to you.

I might add that I know, in your quest for effective management of an ailing spine, a lot of you will have tried everything. Many a well-intentioned friend or acquaintance will have his or her own bit of advice which he or she will swear by. If you were to take up any one of these suggestions, one might be invaluable, another as helpful as fanning with a straw hat. The variety is limitless. Eventually you will have come across every imaginable suggestion of cure and will have become wearily sceptical of any bright new promises.

It also must be said that the very fact that there exists such a variety of alternatives points an incriminating finger at the medical profession, which has not come up with the one fail-safe way of fixing painful backs.

WHAT WILL TRACTION DO?

Traction is 'the rack'. It consists of a harness around the chest and another one around the hips attached to a variable weight. The patient lies relaxed on the back and the weight pulls or, rather, eases the spinal sections apart. In the absence of more localised and accurate treatment techniques, traction can be the treatment of choice.

However, traction is very inaccurate or non-specific in its action. It simply pulls all the vertebrae apart, so that healthy joints as well as unhealthier tighter joints are included in the treatment. A joint that is very stiff and that may have been stiff for twenty years (which is very common) will hardly be

30 Low lumbar traction.

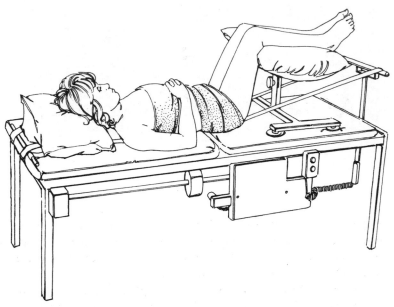

touched by the generalised pull of traction. It does not do the healthier joints any harm to be distracted (separated) — indeed, it probably gives them a bit of a tune-up, which is all very beneficial — but you have not sought help to have your healthy joints treated and the troublemaker ignored.

Even so, traction does have some good uses. I tend to use it rather as a 'fall-back' technique to resort to if my continual handling of a problem joint in the course of treatment has made you sore. This is a common phenomenon and is referred to as treatment soreness (see 'Can Treatment Make Me Worse?' later in the chapter). Here, traction applied in a gentle rhythmical pull-and-release way is very helpful in dispersing bruising while still allowing the process of releasing the joint to continue. It is an effective indirect way of keeping things moving.

Traction is also useful in treating a severely swollen joint which occurs when it is acutely inflamed. When a joint is literally too painful to be touched, it becomes locked in swollen rigidity. Movement causes pain but, paradoxically, because it cannot be moved, the pain gets worse. The circulation in and out of the joint slows down through lack of movement and the tissues become engorged. The joint will be tense and painful.

Normal to-and-fro movement of a healthy functioning joint acts like a pump by shunting blood in and out of a joint. It greatly boosts joint circulation. Without that movement, the blood-flow becomes sluggish and more swelling collects.

In this instance, extremely gentle rhythmic oscillatory traction (2–3 kilo pull or less) will encourage the joint to work normally again. The gentle pull and release of the traction for a brief period of time probably sets up a temporary artificial pump which is sufficient to establish a better filling-and-emptying blood-flow through the soft tissues of the joint, which persists even after the traction is released.

Static traction, which is a continuous distractive pull, can also be used to decongest a severely swollen joint. Here again the weight of the pull is minimal. The effects in this instance are derived from the distraction of the two opposing bony surfaces. The sustained reduction of pressure within the joint for a short period of time (five minutes) is sufficient to allow the tissues time to 'empty' themselves of their stagnant collection of used blood, whereafter more new blood can be pumped in and normal dynamic circulation is restored.

We physios run into trouble when we give the patient in this case too heavy or too long a pull. It is then possible that pulling the joint apart can achieve the converse of what we are trying to do. The joint becomes engorged and bloated by the pooling of blood in the joint's soft tissues. If this were to happen, you would feel much worse as soon as the traction were released. You would barely be able to get off your back, and you would wonder what on earth had been done to you. There is no other option but to go straight on to the traction table again and over a period of time — say, an hour or so — have the weight of the pull gradually reduced. We have all done this to someone at least once in a lifetime, and I tell you it is hell. That patient cannot get out of there quickly enough.

Traction of a very different kilo pull (over 40 kilos) is very useful in treating the non-painful, chronically stiff back with bad degenerative change present at every level. In these cases the physio has to call up every technique in the book to get some movement in that stiff, prematurely old back.

Traction will be used in combination with vigorous manual mobilisation, treading on the spine — indeed, dancing on the spine (with you lying on the floor and me hanging on to the treatment couch for stability) — and an elaborate variety of stretching exercises as a home regime for you to do between each treatment session.

I am frequently asked whether hanging from the doorway has any therapeutic value. It does. The only problem is that you have such a hard job holding on grimly with the fingers that it is hardly relaxed enough to be beneficial. Many

The direction of the distractive force of traction

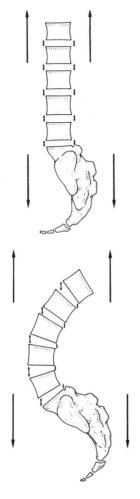

31 If the spine is subjected to a distractive force while it is curved, there is an unequal pull across partially opened joints.

people say that it is exactly what they feel the back needs. Then I am in full agreement because I am a great believer in the directives of intuition. And, besides, it might do some good. But if a joint is pulled apart when it is partially hinged there is a disproportionate pull with the open side being more stretched than the closed side. Traction is most effective therefore when the joint is in mid-position. If you have a low lumbar problem, try to take the hollow out of your back as you hang there; if the pain is higher up in the low back, try to arch as you hang there.

I am also asked about 'Backswing' frames, those contraptions which snap around your ankles and allow you to hang upside down, relaxed and floppy, so that the vertebrae can pull apart. Benefit is directly proportional to the degree of relaxation. In general they are moderately effective but, again, their disadvantage is that the maximum distraction takes place where there is minimal curve of the spine, which means at the upper lumbar level. If you have a high lumbar problem, then they are excellent, but most problems are lower and barely benefit from this sort of pull.

BACKBLOCK

But there IS another way of getting the lower vertebral segments of the spine to separate, which is a whole lot easier and more accurate than hanging upside down; not to mention cheaper. This employs the use of the BackBlock, a humble device based upon an Iyengar yoga concept. To me the BackBlock is living proof of the principle: simple is genius. Who would have thought that a chunk of wood, something so perfectly unpretentious, could be more helpful than just about anything else for an ailing spine? Except for thumbs that is.

Because our spine carries itself upright, over time the lower end tends to telescope into itself. If you imagine the movements of the spine as resembling a vertical concertina which sinks and springs under the effects of gravity with every movement we make, it is not too hard to imagine that the lower segments will bunch up. This is a fundamental truism of the maturing human spine. With the vertical compression of the column, the bricks at the bottom of the stack jam down closer on one another, because of all the super-incumbent weight. Just as if the base of the spine were caught in a vice, everything is pressed together. Opposing bony surfaces of neighbouring vertebrae press together, the discs flatten as fluid is squeezed out, binding soft tissues pucker as the spine shortens its length, so that overall, fluid movement becomes leaden movement. The spine feels brittle and jerky as it rolls and flips around itself in normal activity.

The business of sitting potentiates all this. The added compression of sitting bunches up the base even more. And remember, Western man sits all the time, ramming his butt up under the base of his spine – driving, eating, reading, writing, telephoning, sewing, typing, watching television. Like the concertina where one end cannot be pulled out, the bottom end of our spine never gets a chance to drop down and disengage. We are all walking around with permanently jammed up lower spines. Human beware.

But there is another set of factors which further predispose the base of the human spine to trouble. This is all to do with the fact that we do everything bent. Our activity mode is always one of crumple. As we concentrate our gaze over the task at hand, we curl forward. This is so whether we are sitting, say threading a needle, or standing raking the leaves or maybe bending over shearing a sheep.

This predominance of one-way activity has long term effects on the skeleton as a whole; we develop a stoop. Even if it isn't an obvious stoop, as a dynamic phenomenon we lose the ability to go back the other way; to arch backwards. This permanent state of imbalance, superimposed on the impacted brittleness of the lower spine means that problems of spinal function are just beneath the surface. The back is easy to hurt and sooner or later there will be pain.

This is where the BackBlock comes in. It undoes both sets of problems. It is an oblong of wood about half the thickness of a shoe box which you lie over backwards.

Here is the way to do it. Begin by lying on your back on the floor. With your knees bent, lift up your pelvis and slide the block of wood in under your bottom. It should fit quite comfortably there under the sacrum, that hard flat bone at the base of the spine where the two dimples in the lower back indicate the joints on either side. From here, one at a time, allow both legs to straighten out along the floor and relax. Try to keep both heels together though your feet will roll out. You must completely "let go" and there will be a sensation of agreeable discomfort, a pulling-out feeling in the lower back and across the front of the hips. Don't be alarmed that you feel a certain degree of unease, even pain of the familiar nature you have long complained of. That sweet pain will always be associated with a sense of sweet release. It goes right to the nub of things and usually causes you to feel a specific local

1 Lie on back on floor, knees bent, Lift bottom, slide block at flattest, crossways, under the hard, flat bone at base of spine. Straighten one leg at a time out along the floor so that both legs are flopped, heels together. Remain as long as possible: this may only be a few seconds

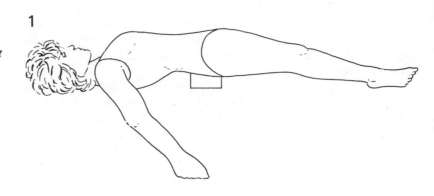

2 After coming off block, always gather one knee up with the hand and gently bounce on the chest. Repeat with the other leg. Lie flat on the floor and relax for a minute or two. Turn on to the right side before getting up.

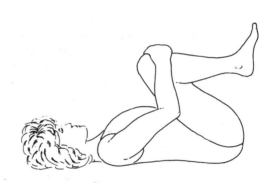

3 Progress by turning block on to long edge, crossways, Increase time from 30 seconds as discomfort eases. Lift off and relax to floor between times. Note: It often hurts to lift your weight off the block. Don't panic. Repeat Procedure 2.

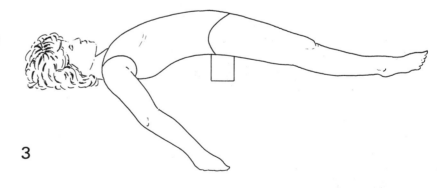

discomfort, right at the source of things, where you know something to be amiss.

The action of lying backwards passively over the block, gently opens out the low back; just like sucking out a concertina. Of all the myriad movements you have performed in your life, this action you have probably never done. It is remarkable that by just lying there, gravity separates the jammed lower vertebrae

4

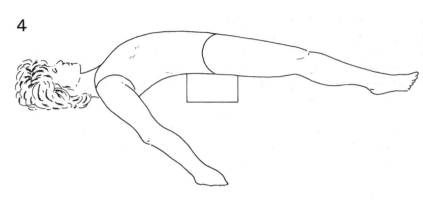

4 Progress by turning the block, long edge lengthwise, under the hard, flat sacrum. As discomfort eases, increase the time 30 seconds to 10 minutes with breaks between. Repeat Procedure 2.

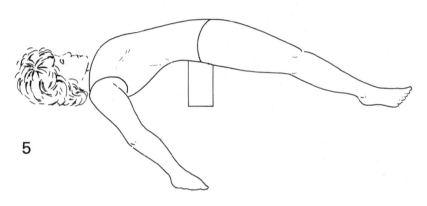

5

5 Only for the very fit! Stand block on end. Progress times as before. It may take several weeks, even months, to progress through each successive phase. Repeat Procedure 2.

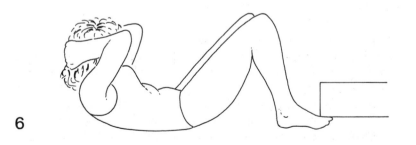

6

6 FOR ALL BLOCK POSITIONS: After coming off block and bouncing knees, do some gentle sit-ups with feet secured. Progress up from 5 to a maximum of 30, the longer the time on the block the more sit-ups. If difficult, pull up with hands on thighs, return to floor with hands behind head, as shown. Curl up, roll down.

and also takes you out of your habitual stoop. It is a magic combination; and so simple. Of course you can do similar backward arching in the prone lying position as shown in Diagram 40.4 and in the standing position as shown in Diagram 40.5. But in both these procedures, although you get the benefit of the backward arch, you fail to get the traction or pulling apart of the lower-most vertebrae. Indeed you even get

* WARNING Do not attempt to use the BackBlock if you feel pain or strain or if you knowingly have a back disorder.

the reverse; greater impaction than ever, which in some instances is undesirable.

The BackBlock can be utilised in progressive stages. First of all on its flattest side so that your bottom rests only five or so centimetres off the floor. Once you have mastered that, by lying over it for longer and longer periods (up to ten or fifteen minutes), you will progress to lying over it on its longest edge, running across-ways under your sacrum, which raises you about 12 centimetres off the floor and increases the arch. Again, do this for longer and longer periods. The next advance is to turn the block, still on the same edge, lengthwise under your sacrum. This is a much narrower surface of support which allows the two sacro-iliac joints at either side of the sacrum, to join in the stretch. Eventually, some very lax-jointed types can even progress to using it on its end. But this is not to be entered into with flippant abandon.

Simple as the BackBlock routine sounds, it is often astonishingly uncomfortable to persevere with, certainly in the beginning. Some people, even those without a back problem, cannot remain up on the flattest edge for longer than a few seconds. (They, incidentally have problems in store.) This quickly improves as one slides the block out, returns to the floor, does some knees to chest bounces, and then tries again.

I have taken to supplying these BackBlocks to all my patients. I provide them complete with transfers of explanations and progressive mode of use, simply because they make my job so much easier. You can achieve a similar result by lying over a couple of telephone books, but unfortunately, this arrangement lacks the wherewithal to be progressed in the same manner. With the BackBlocks, I ask people to use theirs every day. I even use one myself, watching the television news over it every evening. I stay on it for a minute or two, going off it when it gets too uncomfortable and back on it again after I have loosened up with a few knees bounces to the chest. Such a relief incidentally, to derive so much benefit from so little effort. None of this work ethic stuff of progress only through grit.

The only important rejoinder to be made about the use of the BackBlock is that curl-ups must ALWAYS follow. And it is imperative that you never lapse. The sequence is: BackBlock then curl-ups. The longer the time on the block, the more the number of curl-ups (up to about 30). If you find that you are rather stiff after you have come off the block (and this is quite common), precede the curl-ups with leisurely bounces of the knees to the chest, as shown in Diagram 43.1, firstly one at a time and then both together. This loosens things up enough to allow the curl-ups to be done painlessly.

SHOULD I NOT REST IN BED?

Rest in bed is really cheating. The rationale is straightforward enough. If one does not know what the matter is, or what else to do, then rest in bed will do no harm. Meanwhile you hope that whatever is wrong will conveniently go away.

If the problem is lack of mobility of a joint — the most common back problem — then rest in bed is about the last thing it needs; that is, if you are hoping to cure yourself of the disability once and for all. It will simply allow the joint to get stiffer and the problem to become more intractable.

Although it is true that the brief spell in a horizontal position may ease your present symptoms, the causal problem of poor segmental function has not been dealt with. By remaining untreated it will sit there ready to complain again at the earliest opportunity, just as soon as it is provoked by an awkward movement.

However, there are some instances where rest in bed is the ideal course of action. One is where a joint is so irritable that even the slightest movement will bring on angry, even unbearable pain. Physical treatment — that is, passively mobilising the joint — will at this stage only make matters worse. Better to rest completely. This even means bedpans instead of going to the lavatory, so that the acute inflammation can die down.

The bed must be firm; you must lie completely flat with only one pillow, never in a half-sitting position, bolstered up with cushions. However, in that bed you may move around as much as you like. All body movements help, especially wriggling movements.

Another instance where bed rest is used is that of a severe intervertebral disc protrusion. If surgery is indicated but the sufferer is unwilling, then the only way of relieving the stretch on the nerve is rest. There is a chance at this stage that it will buy time for the disc to shrink. This means spending about three weeks or more lying flat. It is hoped that by not imposing weight on the disc the weakness of the disc wall will heal and therefore cease bulging when you are upright again.

I prefer to believe that in such cases most improvement is brought about by the spontaneous settling of the inflammation of the nearby soft tissues, and that it is the general inflammation, not simply the pressure from the disc, which is inflaming the nerve.

But in fact a good rest in bed does everything some good. It provides a much needed respite from the ordeal. It temporarily removes you from the chaos of running a work-life while trying to endure intolerable pain. It allows you time to recover a bit of energy, all reserves being depleted by the fight against pain; it allows time for the disc to shrink; it allows time for the general all-round inflammation in the area to die down.

CAN MASSAGE HELP A PAINFUL BACK?

Massage is very nice, but it only indirectly helps backpain.

Massage fails to get into the fundamental problem of the underlying joint performance. It may certainly give temporary relief, and nobody minds that; but, if you want the problem fixed, massage will not do that.

When a spinal joint is irritable the overlying spinal muscles will automatically go into an involuntary 'protective muscle spasm'. This spasm is in itself uncomfortable, like a low-grade cramp. Its purpose is temporarily to 'splint' the hurt joint so that it is not excessively moved again before it can take the strain. Sometimes this muscle spasm becomes extreme, beyond that which one might expect in the circumstances. This often happens because you are so frightened that you add your own 'optional' muscle tenseness to the already-present automatic spasm. These muscles feel sore and tender to touch, but it must be remembered that they are only in a state of spasm because a joint nearby is in trouble. To treat the muscle spasm with massage is to treat the effect and to ignore the cause.

Like all things, though, there are times when the opposite is true, when massage to the muscles alone will have great therapeutic benefit. I need briefly to describe how muscles work and the differing roles of the two main types of skeletal muscle to explain how massage might be useful as a form of treatment.

Muscles are composed of muscle fibres which clump together side by side. The genius factor which makes them muscles and not other soft tissues such as tendons and ligaments is that muscles can contract and shorten in length. Take the biceps muscle, for example, which spans the elbow. At a given message from the brain, all the individual biceps muscle fibres shorten themselves and pull in the muscle's length. The magic this performs is to bend the elbow. Because the shortening process always happens across a joint, the joint is caused to bend. All muscles work in this way and they all have their own joint to work on. They act like pulleys working levers (the bones) and this is how the jointed skeleton moves our bodies in the beautifully synchronised streamlined way which we see every day and take for granted.

Broadly speaking, there are two basic groups of muscles which interact to make the skeleton function purposefully. The first are the antigravity muscles which are in action the entire time and keep the skeleton poised in an upright stance, making all the background positional adjustments to set the stage for all the other whimsical phasic functions we might choose to do. The muscles in the antigravity group are large muscles with coarse strong fibres — for example, the quadriceps muscles which brace the knees and prevent them from buckling as we stand there. Another group is the gluteal muscles, the muscles of the bottom, which contract all the time and keep us from folding up at the hips. A further important group is the long strap-like muscles of the spine which keep the torso from slumping forward.

Smaller, more delicate phasic muscles perform all those other transient, elective motions that make up the living person, be it bringing a spoon to the mouth, smiling or tapping the foot to music.

The important thing to be stressed is that the first group is on duty all the time — unlike the muscles of the second group, which come into play only to make a fleeting appearance and then withdraw. For example, you might be roused to smile broadly. Your head is already in position, sitting up fair and square above your shoulders as a matter of course, because the muscles in the back of the neck are keeping it there all the time you are up and awake. You do not have to exert any will over them, even though you might over the muscles that make a smile.

Antigravity muscles therefore have a laborious job. They operate by keeping up a monotonous state of low-grade contraction, quite unlike the phasic ones, which burst into action with a great flurry of activity and when it is all over settle back in comfort and relax.

The job of the antigravity muscles is made even more laborious if the postural alignment of the skeleton is so bad that they must work overtime simply to keep the skeleton upright and poised for action. This overwork demanded of the muscles is very taxing. Over a period of time it causes them to lose the ability to relax, even after their role is no longer required.

Such sustained, heightened contraction of the muscles is known as chronic spasm. If spasm is particularly relentless, some of the muscle fibres change in nature, losing their original qualities of contractability. The muscle develops hard tender cords and is said to be 'fibrositic'. This is not a common cause of low backache; it is more usually a problem across the back of neck and shoulders, the chronic spasm in this case being the outcome of a head perpetually carried too far forward. The overworked trapezius muscle is always trying to pull it back in line with the rest of the spine, and failing.

Massage of the fibrositis helps to break down the hard lumps and render the tissues softer. This will make the muscles more comfortable, but permanent relief will only be gained by loosening the joints of the neck and thorax and establishing a better posture so that the strain disappears. But the massage in this case must be deep and painful to break down the knots.

Another ideal application for massage is to promote relaxation. It is true that, in the presence of chronic backpain, lack of relaxation, that is, tension, will increase the pain (see 'Does Tension Make My Back Worse?' Chapter 8). Therefore, if generalised body massage will bring about an all-round reduced state of anxiety/tension, then that is surely desirable. In this case the massage can be gentle or hard, whichever proves the more relaxing.

WHAT WILL PILLS DO?

There are three groups of tablets which help you cope with the problem of pain, but do not expect too much from the pill-bottle. With a simple back problem unrelated to disease, no tablet will get rid of the underlying disturbance of function which is the cause of the pain.

Painkillers or Analgesics

Provided that you are undergoing physical treatment to undo the mechanical problem, there is no harm in making yourself a little more comfortable for the duration. Painkillers are useful just to knock the peak off the pain, especially if that pain has been temporarily increased by the treatment itself.

So far as choice of drugs is concerned, there is one golden

rule: Always follow prescribed dosages. This may be saying the obvious with prescription-only drugs such as codeine, but the rule applies with equal force to ordinary over-the-counter drugs such as aspirin or paracetamol.

Muscle Relaxants

As a natural automatic reflex, when a joint or disc is causing trouble, the overlying back muscles will go into protective muscle spasm to try to protect that segment from immediate further assault. These muscles are the caretakers of the joint. After a relatively brief period of time, once the muscles perceive that the joint is able to move slightly without too much alarm, the muscle spasm fades away. If you are in a heightened anxiety state, or if the trauma sustained by the segment is fairly severe, the muscle spasm remains intense and intractable. The sooner that muscle spasm can be eliminated the better. It aggravates the hurt joint to have it remain jammed by the overlying muscle spasm. Furthermore, treatment for the actual joint is held up while the muscle spasm is dealt with by the drugs. Muscle in spasm is also painful in its own right and as such is another source of pain.

Muscle relaxants help ease muscle spasm. They make the muscle caretakers sleepy and less vigilant. By reducing their hold, they allow the segment to begin making its first tentative movements again. The pain-free movement indicates to the muscles that the cause for alarm has passed and their over-energetic attendance is no longer required.

Anti-Inflammatory Drugs

Any joint that is not working properly is by nature 'inflamed'. The degree of inflammation varies, but the pain increases as the degree of inflammation increases. Anti-inflammatory drugs act directly on the inflammatory process to quell it. They also act to minimise the pain of treatment soreness when therapy has of necessity been aggressive and lengthy because the joint stiffness is proving difficult to undo.

There are a number of anti-inflammatory drugs that may be prescribed for backpain. Some, such as aspirin and indomethacin, have analgesic properties as well. Most, if not all, anti-inflammatory drugs have some side-effects. If you experience these even on a low dosage, you should ask to try another sort of compound. The side-effects I am thinking of are stomach pains, diarrhoea, nausea, dizziness and headaches. High blood-pressure and pregnancy do not mix well with certain anti-inflammatory agents. You should never indiscriminately swallow any medication upon your own initiative. You should closely follow your doctor's orders. You should never commence or cease taking medication during a course of treatment, because this will give an unrealistic reading on the progress of treatment.

SHOULD I HAVE SPINAL INJECTIONS?

In cases of severe back or leg pain which is highly irritable to physical treatment and is not responding to rest in bed or tablets, either, it is often of great value to inject a local dose of cortico-steroid (a fairly powerful anti-inflammatory agent) into the spine itself, to act on the inflammation directly.

The spinal cord is the soft squashy bundle of nerve pathways running down the inside of the spinal column from the base of the brain. Spinal nerves branch off all the way down the cord to leave the spine at each intervertebral level. The cord and its branches float in fluid inside a loose sack, the sack having continuous 'sleeves' clothing the nerves until they are clear of the bony channels through which they leave the spine. This membranous sack is called the 'dura'.

An epidural injection squirts local anaesthetic and cortisone into the inside of the spinal column, stopping short of the sack, that is, without puncturing it, and in effect bathes the dura in this local medication. It is effective in quelling the inflammation of the nervous tissue and the sack or sheath and thus reducing the pain. It may only take effect after making the pain worse for one or two days.

There is a branch of manipulative medicine which believes in the use of 'sclerosant' or 'sclerosin' injections. These are a sugar compound which by irritating the soft tissues after injection are said to cause scar tissue formation which binds up a loose and over-wobbly joint, and reduces symptoms caused by that unstable joint. Some practitioners appear to use sclerosants on all types of back problem, loose joints and stiff joints alike. They claim that this is of benefit to many back sufferers. But I wonder whether it may not be the 'placebo' effect or perhaps the counter-irritation effect whereby an 'old' pain is replaced temporarily by a 'new' pain of slightly different nature, thence blocking permanently the old pain pathway.

I do not know if these injections work; or, if they do work, why they work.

DO I NEED AN OPERATION?

A surgical operation on the spine may be advised in those circumstances where there has been unbearable pain (particularly leg pain) over a long period of time, unrelieved or made worse by manual treatment; where there are advanced and progressive neurological signs (such as loss of reflexes, numbness, pins and needles, loss of muscle power, and disturbance of sensation of the saddle area with difficulty in passing urine).

There are two main operations for a bad back.

One is the laminectomy. This involves removing the disc and some of the nearby bone, by picking away at the bony canal down which the nerve travels on its way to the outside of the spine after it has branched off the spinal cord floating inside the spine. This operation is not as drastic as it might seem. It does not weaken the spine's mechanical strength at all. It simply widens the bore of the canal, along which the spinal nerve leaves the spine.

The prime consideration, therefore, after the first twenty-four hours following surgery, after all the bleeding has stopped, is to get the spine moving again. Movement is not dangerous.

The complications after laminectomy are often brought about by failure to get up and going soon enough after surgery. The reason for this is that, with prolonged inactivity after a bleed into tissues, blood tends to lie around and stagnate. It needs instead to be shunted away by the normal pumping action created by natural movements.

If you remain inactive, this blood and fluid in time tends to become thicker and more gelatinous. It starts to clog up the delicate spinal machinery. If inactivity persists, this substance gets even thicker so that, eventually, it becomes scar tissue, or 'adhesions', which is simply non-specific living junk. If you do not make deliberate efforts to get moving, that useless material really takes hold. It gets in around the nerve root which has just been surgically freed and brings about the very symptoms you have just had surgery to rectify.

It is important to stress that you need not expect to have a permanently handicapped spine after a laminectomy. Although there is an impressive long scar left behind after

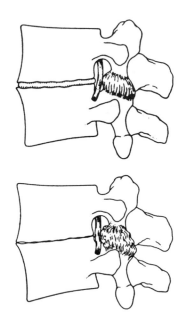

32 Grumbling facet joint trouble can be aggravated by joint-surface jamming after removal of a disc.

surgery, the intrinsic strength of the back has in no way been impaired. There is absolutely no need for you to creep about as if your back is going to break!

The unfortunate and unwelcome recurrence of the same degree of backpain after surgery or even more severe sciatic pain after surgery has caused many a furrowed brow and sad shake of the head. However, it leads me again to make the assumption that the disc was not causing the symptoms in the first place. It points the finger very definitely to the facet joint as the perpetrator of the mischief.

If the pain indeed worsens after surgery, I suspect that a facet joint problem has been stirred up by the effects of the surgery. The simplest explanation is that as soon as the patient is upright and walking about after the operation the two opposing surfaces of the problem facet joint, formerly kept apart by the presence of a robust disc, become jammed together (see diagram 32). The backpain will worsen.

However, as mentioned earlier, it is also true that scar tissue may proliferate to an inordinate degree after surgery and this also may be a reason for an increase in pain following it. The amount of scar tissue produced depends on both the delicacy of the operative procedure and the inherent tendency of some individuals to produce heavy scarring. The scar tissue causes trouble when it infiltrates around the cord and the nerve roots and re-creates pressure, even though the disc has been removed.

The development of sciatic pain resulting from scar tissue formation is slower and more insidious — say, six weeks as the scar develops — than in the case of a jammed facet joint, when there is likely to be almost instantaneous recurrence of pain after surgery as soon as the patient gets upright.

There is another variation in the picture of pain which persists after surgery, but in this instance it *is* the disc which caused the sciatic pain. One commonly sees in practice that the operation gets rid of the more recent leg pain but fails to get rid of the original backache. A common pattern with a progressively troublesome back is that backpain of several years' origin later develops into backpain plus leg pain or sciatica. This happens because the disc eventually starts to bulge as a final stage of degeneration of the whole spinal segment, the sequence of which has been described earlier. The bulge squashes the spinal nerve and causes leg pain. The erstwhile simple picture of common or garden backache arising from rusty facet joints of the spine has developed into a more complicated picture of two pains arising from two different sources, the facet joint and the disc, together as the problem gets worse. Surgery at this stage may relieve you only of the secondary problem but it will fail to relieve you of the original facet joint problem. In fact, it will probably intensify it.

The second common operative procedure for a bad back is the spinal fusion. This is simply the surgical joining of one vertebra to another and is indicated when too much movement has developed at an intervertebral level. That level then becomes unstable and is unable to be sufficiently stabilised by strengthening exercises (see Chapter 6).

Sometimes fusions are performed after the laminectomy, in the course of the same operation. It may be thought that removal of a troublesome intervertebral disc would bring about a new sloppiness at the operated level. Beforehand, though being a cause of trouble, the disc had at least by its very width kept its two adjacent vertebrae well sprung apart and therefore the spine tightly functional. Removal of that disc might well bring about a 'new' internal weak link in the spine.

Fusion at this stage may also be done to ease a severe inflammation of a segment. By obliterating all movement, the inflammation will settle.

The drawback with spinal fusion is that to obliterate movement at a spinal level does eventually cause other problems elsewhere later on. The lack of movement of a fused segment must be compensated for by over-movement somewhere else, at some level above or below the fused one. It is almost impossible for this helpful joint to tolerate the added load indefinitely without strain. After several years, if not before, the compensation joint will start to show signs of irritation caused by excessive movement, and this joint, too, will become a problem joint.

The other developmental problem of a spinal fusion is the insidious progressive choking of the spinal nerves as they issue out of the spine, under the fused part. As we saw earlier, normal movement begets normal joints. Normal movement keeps a joint free, streamlined, efficient and uncongested. The reverse is true in a joint where movement has been artificially blocked. For example, even in the absence of injury or disease of the hand, normal healthy fingers which are kept immobile for a couple of days will puff up like little sausages. This happens simply because the pumping action of muscular activity has been stopped. As a result the circulation slows and the digits fill up with fluid. (It is for this reason, incidentally, that broken fingers these days are never splinted in plaster of Paris to allow the fracture to heal. They are simply strapped to a neighbouring healthy finger so that as the bone mends the joint keeps moving. We do this because we now know that the stiffness developed in the small finger joints is a much greater complication in the long term than the broken bone.)

During the operative procedure for spinal fusion, as for the laminectomy, there is a lot of surgical cutting of the tissues. Blood and clear lymph fluid oozes out. This lies about in the tissues between the muscles and ligaments and stagnates. Because the joint has been splinted rigid by two large metal screws joining one vertebra to another, this fluid will not be naturally dispersed by movement and carried away by the bloodstream. There exists a backwater, or stasis of circulation, around the fusion — the first step in the formation of 'adhesions'.

These adhesions, or scar tissue, may become so prolific that they severely clutter the small channels in which the spinal nerves make their exit. The channels become choked and the nervous tissue becomes physically thwarted by this undergrowth of living invasive junk.

Another complication of fusion — and of laminectomy, too, for that matter — is excessive new bone growth. This happens where the top hard layer of bone is bevelled away by a surgical chisel in the course of the operative technique. Denuded of its top hard layer, new bone growth tends to proliferate. This, too, gets in the way of the nerves.

This insidious development of prolific scar tissue or new bone growth or both may not necessarily irritate the spinal nerve too much because both are fairly benign. You would not, as a matter of course, get normal old backpain. However, it may so squeeze the nervous tissue that it may restrict its very blood supply, and this means trouble.

In its normal healthy state, the spinal cord and its branches, the spinal nerves, have such an abundant blood supply that, when they are exposed at surgery, they pulsate with blood as each successive pulse-wave shunts through. A fine lacework of blood vessels climb all over a nerve, around and through the nervous tissue, and keep it adequately supplied with generous quantities of good, clean, health-giving blood. The supply is quickly increased upon demand, that demand being created by an escalation of muscle activity. When the blood supply is constricted by bony or fibrous entrapment within either the spinal canal or the nerve root canal, the flow of blood with each pulse beat is reduced to a meagre trickle. When the area is exposed at operation, the pulsation of blood coursing through the vascular network is no longer obvious to the naked eye.

When extra work is demanded of the nerves — particularly, say, when you climb a hill or walk up stairs — they suffer what is known as vascular embarrassment. You will experience a particularly nasty pain in the leg which rapidly intensifies as the walking continues. This syndrome is called spinal stenosis.

The pain in the leg is not dissimilar to the cramps caused by circulatory problems. The steeper the slope, the worse the pain. The only way to relieve the pain is to stop walking. You feel an irresistible desire to sit down or to squat. The curled position widens the diameter of the spinal canal, all fuzzed up with useless tissue clutter, and allows the nerve more room in which to get a surging blood supply through.

Stenosis can develop after surgery because of proliferation of bone growth as a result of the top layer of bone being chiselled away. All bone is in fact soft tissue in a very hard form. Like all soft tissue, it weeps after trauma and then replaces itself in the healing process with bony 'callus'. The bone always produces more callus than is needed. So whether it be repair after breaking a leg or after a surgeon has been scraping away with a chisel an excess of bone will appear at the site of action. This can be disastrous inside the spine because there is not enough room for any more space-occupying matter as well as the nerve. The nerve gets squashed by the new growth. Hence spinal stenosis.

Developmental stenosis, when it occurs, is a very difficult state of affairs to rectify. It is counter-productive to go in again surgically since the same chain of events is almost certain to occur again with even more scar tissue likely to grow next time.

Although most back operations are successful, they are essentially treatment of the last resort. Manual therapy should always be tried as a conservative measure before surgery is contemplated. In the case of spinal stenosis, mobilisation with the fingers does have a small role to play. It is possible to get some breaking down of the adhesions by simply kneading them with deep manual pressure but it is a long job.

SHOULD I TRY ACUPUNCTURE?

It must be said that there are cases where acupuncture succeeds when all else has failed.

I believe acupuncture to be particularly useful in the control of backpain in those cases where, even though the original underlying physical joint problem has been rectified, lingering muscle spasm persists — perhaps because the 'pain memory pathways' in the brain had been so well trodden that the messages continue to be passed, regardless of the need.

It would appear that acupuncture in this instance seems to break the pain circuit. How it does this is not altogether clear. One recent suggestion is that the ancient tradition of inserting needles into various parts of the body — not necessarily those that are giving the pain — may activate the release of special pain-killing substances called 'endorphines', thereby dampening down pain. But our knowledge is sketchy and highly speculative, especially mine.

WHAT IS MANIPULATION?

Manipulation is the therapeutic cracking of a joint with a quick thrust or tug. Although it is a gentle delicate procedure, it is so quick and deft that it is impossible for the patient to prevent the manoeuvre from taking place.

In theory, it is sudden manual over-pressure at limit of range of movement of a stiff joint to force the joint further towards its expected normal limit of range.

If you manipulate well, you are almost born to manipulate well. It is possible to learn and know the theory of manipulation, but without a natural aptitude you will never do it with great finesse. Osteopaths and chiropractors pioneered the field of manipulative medicine and still today, on balance, probably accomplish the manoeuvres with greater flair and aplomb than the average physiotherapist.

Only relatively recently has manipulation been looked upon more favourably by conservative medicine. It was originally viewed as a dangerous fringe practice, which inevitably forced it further into the realms of the crank, with a lot of lay manipulators practising freely.

Manipulation is not dangerous if the patient is healthy. Stories of disasters propagated by gleeful scaremongers were usually incidents where there were other medical conditions which went undiagnosed before the treatment began, such as rheumatoid arthritis or bone tumours. Manipulation should not bear the blame. The skeleton with its elastic ligaments holding its joints together is pretty resilient. Routine clinical investigations carried out by a doctor before the patient is sent for physiotherapy will sift out those patients unsuitable for manipulation.

Manipulation usually produces a characteristic popping or cracking sound. There have been many proposals put forward as to what actually makes the sound. My view is that it is caused by the suction effect created by suddenly pulling apart two joint surfaces which had hitherto hung together at a slight negative pressure inside the joint capsule. Others contend that it is the formation and collapse of a gas bubble in a hundredth of a second that is responsible for the crack. It is definitely not the breaking or tearing of adhesions nor the sound of bones being put back into place. Furthermore, there is absolutely no foundation whatsoever for the claim that the cracking sound is the sucking back and repositioning of a 'slipped disc'.

When a disc is in trouble it is because the nucleus has bulged over to one side of the disc causing its wall to balloon out. It has been long established that this process never takes place instantly. It happens over a period of time as the disc's health deteriorates.

As we spend most of our time working either bent over or sitting down, the lumbar spine slumps and the discs are all squashed out at the back. After a period of time the nucleus starts to squirt through the inner layers of the retaining rim of the disc: it is no longer able to tolerate and disperse the pressure of the weight it is subjected to.

It is therefore unrealistic to expect that one yank on the poor disc can persuade the nucleus to go back to the centre. It would be rather like trying to push toothpaste back into its tube, and then failing to screw the cap on. Even if it were possible to reposition the nucleus, to expect the split in the cartilage then miraculously and instantaneously to mend over when cartilage has no blood supply and takes months to regenerate anyway is asking too much.

As comforting as that crack is, the fact of the matter is that it has no significant therapeutic value at all. Healthier joints do crack more readily than unhealthy ones, and the only relevance of the noise is that in the early stages of treatment the joint will probably not crack when manipulated, but as the joint performance improves later on in the treatment it will crack with manipulation. The manipulation is just as effective without the crack as with it. But it takes some doing to convince a patient of that.

WHAT IS MOBILISATION?

Ah, the crucial question!

The concept of manual joint mobilisation (Maitland Mobilisation) is the evolution of the life and work of Geoffrey D. Maitland, physiotherapist of Adelaide, South Australia. He developed the concept from his technical skill with his hands together with his knowledge of the other branches of manipulative medicine, coalesced over the years into a carefully designed management of faulty joints. I am a non-purist disciple of Maitland. I have picked up a lot of his ideas and mixed them with a mash of my own.

So we manual therapists are joint specialists. Joint performance is our speciality; not only spinal joints, but the peripheral joints as well, like shoulders, knees, jaws, etc., etc.

Joints are a dynamic system; they are temperamental and prone to dysfunction, and they give the skeleton much more aggravation than the bones do!

To break a bone always arouses alarm. Well, the bones actually do quite well after being broken. Given time and a bit of splinting to hold the bone fragments together, they knit together in no time and actually end up stronger than they were originally.

However, the joints, too, can be dreadfully mangled and pulled about by the same injury, but because they tolerate such a lot of shock with very little complaint and few outward signs of ill effect, their lowered state of health and reduced performance can easily be overlooked.

Traditionally, stiff joints have never been seen as anything other than stiff joints. They have long escaped the attention of clinical scrutiny because it had not been realised that simple joint malfunction could be capable of causing a lot of pain, directly or indirectly.

The phenomenon of 'referred pain' makes it harder to trace general aches and pains to a particular malfunctioning joint, because it often creates a pain quite far distant from the joint itself. This may have led to the diagnosis of 'fibrositis', 'muscle tear', 'ligament sprain', 'internal bruising', 'blood clot', etc., etc., etc., as some of the many and varied explanations for all sorts of simple aches and pains.

In the process of treating a spine by manual mobilisation we first of all watch the spine performing its major movements and note any deficiencies. We then feel with our hands for the individual mobility of the segments. This is done while you lie face down on the treatment couch — the spine spread out and relaxed, accessible to the investigative probing and pressing from the physio's hands.

Patches of stiffness in the spine are immediately apparent. The block in spinal mobility feels like a plug of cement in a rubber hose. The vertebrae fail to slide away freely under the pressure of the approaching hands. They resist being moved, feeling hard and unyielding to the pressure.

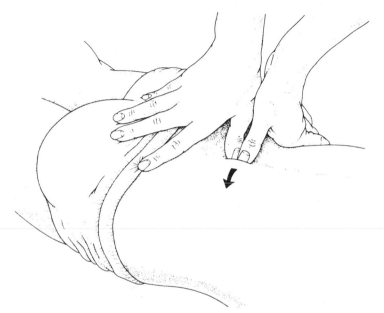

Mobilisation with the thumbs gently eases a stiff vertebra.
33.1 It can be done in a transverse direction so that the vertebra swivels.

You, too, will be aware that something is amiss when such a vertebra is pressured. There is either a local soreness, as if the bone itself is bruised, or perhaps complete reproduction of the familiar backpain that you have so long complained of. To all practical ends it is not imperative to reproduce the exact pain; a comparable discomfort is proof enough that this is where the trouble is.

However, it may be that to reproduce the pain, the spinal segments are quite free to glide forwards and backwards on one another but are completely unable to swivel or glide sideways on one another. This will still constitute a fault of function and it will be a source of pain.

The therapeutic part of the process follows. The therapist's thumbs find that rusty segment of spine and gently but relentlessly prise it free. This is done with gentle push and release pressures usually with the thumbs, but perhaps with the heel of the hand, the knee, the elbow or even the heel of the foot.

33.2 It can be done in a forwards/ backwards direction so that the vertebra glides back and forth between its neighbours.

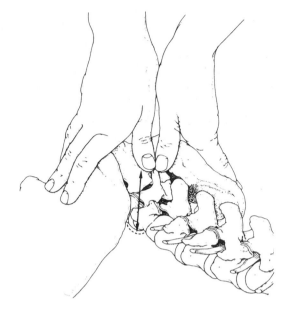

Quite quickly the vertebrae will begin to move again and participate as they should do in total spinal mobility. The length of time it takes to free a stiff segment depends on how long it has taken to get into such a state. It may only take one session if you felt something amiss in the back for the first time yesterday. Or you may need intensive treatment for six weeks with follow-up booster sessions every six months for the rest of your life. It helps to do your own maintenance exercises (see Chapter 6).

The key distinction between manipulation and mobilisation is that mobilisation is geared to the state of soreness and debility of the joint. Treatment is geared to how much pushing it can take. As the joint gets freer and less painful, the pressures are increased. Eventually the vertebra can be pushed into all its positions with completely painless freedom. Manipulation, on the other hand, pushes the joint immediately to its limits regardless of state of health.

The graduation of mobilising pressures varies from breath-takingly light-fingered techniques to extremely heavy-handed stuff. In the case of the latter, actually lying you on the floor and standing — indeed, bouncing — on the area where the block is will be the only way to get the joint going again. The other extreme is very gentle pushing, pulling and gliding where the only problem is that you, the patient, may think that not enough is being done to get you better. This is especially so if you are of the tough breed who believe that unless it is agony is is not doing you any good.

There are very specific reasons for using gentle techniques or hefty ones. The longer I practise, the more I use both extremes. I am always standing on backs.

SHOULD TREATMENT HURT?

Broadly speaking, treatment is designed to get rid of pain and, after that, to get rid of the dysfunction, usually stiffness, which by its presence has caused the pain.

Treatment to get rid of pain is so gentle that it is comforting. You are simply having the joint gently and persuasively coaxed into a bit of movement. As movement returns, severe pain that was always present, even while you were doing nothing, will disappear.

Then we have arrived at the slightly more tricky stage of the treatment where fine judgement is required of the therapist. The pain is now much more bearable, but in order to continue improving the problem and to get rid of the root cause once and for all one has to start tackling the lack of mobility of the joint, too. In effect, the physiotherapist is juggling with two sides of the problem at the same time: reducing the resting inflammation and pain, while at the same time starting to push and tug the joint about to restore its original function, lack of which initially caused the pain. But this treatment in itself can hurt and may cause a new pain — treatment soreness. It should be easy to see why sometimes progress is a bit up and down!

In a way, by physically handling and stretching the joint the physiotherapist is artificially irritating the joint, just gently provoking it so that the body defences rally and send blood rushing to the site of the activity. A good physio will not overdo this forced inflammation. It should just stir things up enough so that you are a little sore with a bruised feeling in the evening following the treatment. When this subsides, you realise a new freedom of the spine with progressively less pain. If you feel that you are being 'overdone', then talk to your therapist about it.

When the back problem is more of a nuisance value than a pain, then one usually finds that the spinal joint is just stiff and hardly sensitive at all. Treatment at this stage is designed to get rid of the stiffness in the joint which by its very presence is a source of irritation but, more important, remains as a focus of future trouble. Then treatment is as hefty as the physiotherapist is strong. In my own clinic sometimes two of us will get on to the spine of a patient. Generally speaking, the more the patient yells the better. The patient may be sore for days after one of these sessions. That is all very good.

CAN I BE OVER-TREATED?

Treatment itself causes its own soreness and since this can mimic the original pain, it is often impossible for you to differentiate between the two. You may think that you are worse or you may think that you still need therapy because you still have pain.

It is common for a patient to be discharged from treatment still suffering some degree of pain; we want to leave you alone and allow time to play its role in settling this man-made pain. It may be necessary for you to return to your physio again in six weeks or so just to make sure that there is indeed nothing left of the original problem and that the temporary pain has also gone.

At the other extreme, your physio may still want to drag you back for treatment long after the time when you last felt pain. Be assured that there is a good reason for this. If it is possible to feel by palpation that the spine still lacks some of its varieties of movement, one should continue until the joint is running smoothly in every direction.

We physios are very interested in what we call 'accessory movement' of joints. When any joint bends — say, for example, the elbow — it is not just a pure hinge movement taking place between the two bones. There is a lot of unseen shuffling and swivelling and gliding between the two bones as well as that main obvious joint movement.

The liberty to do this gives the joint a relaxed floppy feel when it is handled by experienced hands. The joint feels empty and loose. Wonderful! It is healthy. When a joint starts to deteriorate this freedom is the first thing to go. The joint feels tight and hard, and when it is professionally assessed it is loath to go into any of its 'unusual' directions. If the joint is to be put absolutely right, then the therapist must persevere with loosening it until all the full 'play' is back and the joint feels nice and empty again, like a loose bag of bones.

So you might think we are making a lot of fuss about nothing. You can get a cup to the mouth. What is the problem? However, if we do not fully mobilise that elbow, getting back all its movements, including the accessory ones, it will seize up again and you will be back, sooner rather than later, for more treatment. The same applies with the joints of the back.

CAN TREATMENT MAKE ME WORSE?

In many ways, treatment is like scratching a scab to make it heal.

Because treatment provokes a reaction, it is possible in the short term to feel worse. However, your condition may actually be improving. As long as the function of the joint is becoming more normal, any pains, either new or old, will eventually disappear. The problem you must grapple with at this stage is your lack of confidence in the treatment and the person administering it.

If you have not been previously warned and adequately comforted at the time and you drop out from treatment, then inevitably you will feel that the treatment made you worse. Time would have told you that you are better. But sadly some patients are not prepared to wait and see. Perhaps you might go off to a faith healer, and because you feel better in a day or two you think he did the trick. I can tell you this has happened to me more than once.

To sum up this chapter, then. There is a variety of treatments and procedures available for the back sufferer, but the central most effective method is that based on joint mobilisation. The others are ancillary to this.

Whatever form of treatment you are undergoing, make sure that your therapist is fully qualified. Never consult an acupuncturist, for example, without doing a little checking first: on his qualifications, experience, reputation.

By now you will know enough about my own technique — mobilisation — to be able to ascertain from any prospective physio how he or she plans to proceed. Don't drive him or her mad with questions on the phone because that will waste time and get his/her back up. However, with treatment you will know fully what to expect and what is unacceptable practice.

5

BENEFITS OF MOBILISATION

AND MANIPULATION

Mobilisation of a joint is a subtle business. Unlike manipulation, there is no drama. No flamboyant thrusts and flourishes. Although the benefits it confers take longer to be realised, the process is kinder to the joints and the effects are therefore longer lasting.

Unlike the osteopath or chiropractor a physiotherapist will not manipulate the back of every person who walks in the door. We will manipulate only when there are specific indications to do so. We believe that living tissue responds better to the persuasive joint-stretching techniques of mobilisation to free a joint progressively over a period of time, rather than to a sudden quick thrust breaking the joint free of its restriction in an instant.

WHAT WILL MOBILISATION ACHIEVE?

A joint will be painful for one of two reasons. First, if it is a problem that has been with you for some time, it will be painful because it is stiff and it simply hurts to bend through the stiffness. Secondly, it may be painful because it is swollen from a recent injury but otherwise not the slightest bit stiff. The first is a chronic state and the second is the acute state after recent trauma.

There is a third reason as well, a combination of these two: an acute injury superimposed on a previous chronic condition, the commonest state of affairs of all. Chronically stiff joints are much more susceptible to further trauma than healthy elastic joints because they cannot roll with the punches.

All sets of circumstances will be helped by gently moving and working the joint; that is, by mobilising it.

Getting rid of the stiffness of a chronic condition is easy to understand. The same applies to a rusty hinge in a door: work it back and forth and you knock off some of the corrosive scale and it runs more freely.

Getting rid of the pain in a chronic condition, when the joint has become tight, is more complicated to understand. The joint is painful because movements of the joint are stretching and tugging at the stiff capsule and, because it is unyielding, the stretch causes pain.

It is easy enough to get rid of the pain by simply making the capsule and the other soft tissues more elastic so that movement does not provoke that stretch pain. Persuasive mobilising, the manual stretching of a joint, will achieve that end fairly quickly, though it may cause pain in the process.

With recent trauma, a completely fresh or virgin joint is yanked about for the first time and is swollen and very painful. Equally, an old joint which has been stiff for years can be provoked anew, causing a whole lot more inflammation and swelling on top of the pre-existing stiffness. In either case, gentle rhythmic joint movement will get rid of the pain.

The highbrow neurophysiological explanation for this is as follows: the new superimposed nerve messages describing the gentle movement going on to the joint have the effect of blocking or dampening former messages about pain coming from that joint.

The familiar automatic response of vigorously shaking the hand having just smashed the thumb with a hammer helps to describe this mechanism. It feels better if you shake it. Just as if you wrench your knee your first instinctive response is immediately to work the knee back and forth, which makes it feel better. Although you do not know it, the brain is being bombarded with messages about gentle movement in preference to the messages about nasty pain. One message overrides the other.

Physiotherapists manually mobilise a painful joint to try to achieve the same result. Treatment is just a professional waggle of the joint, but geared to the level of a joint's irritability.

Movement also has the wonderful advantage of pumping all the swollen engorgement away from the joint so that it can run more freely. If the joint stays still, it gets more swollen. The action of muscles contracting and releasing around a joint dramatically squeezes blood and waste materials out of the tissues and back into the circulation. The joint loses its puffiness. The less the joint moves, the more painful it gets because the more engorged it becomes.

People are often surprised when I attempt very early mobilisation after injury. It seems to fly in the face of all previously held convictions about the need to rest after recent injuries. As a general rule people rest too much. The earlier you start moving the better. You have to get going very early with movement after an injury. If you rest the part — say, an ankle — for a week before trying to move it, not only will it be more painful in the interim as it flops there, hanging inert between the crutches; it will also be a much longer, more painful job eventually to get it moving. This is because all the fluid lying about in the tissues has had time to 'organise' and is well on the way to becoming hard gristly scar tissue. And all scar tissue must be broken down and softened before it can be absorbed into the bloodstream, otherwise the joint will never run freely again.

You might come into our clinic with a seriously painful back. You can hardly move with the pain. We would lie you down on the treatment couch and ever so gently move the joint which is so tense and swollen and responsible for all that pain. Sure enough, though I have hardly dared move the vertebra for fear of worsening the pain, all going well, the joint will become less painful and you will quite quickly be able to move about more freely.

If I were then to lie you down again and remobilise the affected joint, it would very probably be much less sore. It is not uncommon for the patient to think that I have stealthily switched to treating another level, because it feels so much better. Just simple uncomplicated movement has lifted a lot of the pain, and this is the beginning of the process of treatment by mobilisation of a problem joint.

Once we have dealt with the pain, if it is an old or chronic problem, then the matter of stiffness still remains to be dealt with. In order to render the joint completely problem-free in the future, that stiffness must be reversed or the same pattern of inflammation will repeat itself.

As the stiffness eases and the joint becomes more elastic, the pain lessens. Then the mobilisation pressures increase. This highlights again the fundamental difference between manipulation, which is always carried out at the same strength and speed, and mobilisation, which is carefully graduated in step with the ability of the joint to take the force.

CAN I MOBILISE MY OWN SPINE?

Ideally, yes, but in practice it is not easy to manage.

As simple as the concept of manual spinal mobilisation is, it is very difficult to do on one's self. Believe me, I have tried. It is almost impossible to get one's own fingers into a position to do anything useful and all you do is make the joint sore.

In treatment, after we have located the problem level, both by watching the full spinal movement and by feeling the segmental movement, we then, from differing angles depending in which direction the movement is lacking and at differing strengths depending on the amount of resistance encountered, work that segment free. We may even have to lean on it with full body weight using the heel of the hand, or the knee, or even stand and tread on the stiff patch. So as you can see it is fairly hard to duplicate the same action on yourself.

Of course, general spinal movements of forward/back bending, left/right sideways bending, and twisting left/right do rely on all the individual segments doing the same to bring about the overall major movement. So it is true that these general movements done vigorously and fully to the end of range do help to restore segmental mobility. But there is a tendency for the fitter, more mobile neighbouring joints to supplement the movement deficit instead of the inactive one being roused.

For the best outcome, the individual troublemaker has to be sought out and sorted out by means of a pair of thumbs right in at the site of trouble.

However, there is one especially good way of restoring forward/back segmental freedom yourself, and that is by rolling along the spine (see diagram 54, Chapter 6). This is done by lying on the floor on the back, legs held behind the knees with linked hands, and gently rolling along the length of the spine, making sure to concentrate the rolling on the stiff patch that will feel slightly painful as you roll over it. This is an extremely effective procedure and should be done for a few minutes a couple of times a day. Another version of this exercise, more localised to the lowest two lumbar joints is to roll around the sacrum in a circular fashion. Start from the same position, holding the knees and inscribe a wide circle in the air with your knees. This will press your low back into the carpet as you imagine following the triangular outline of the sacrum around.

The last thing to say about self-mobilisation is on the use of a 'Ma Roller', not always available everywhere but excellent for the self-treatment of a low-back problem. They are rather like a convoluted rolling-pin. Made out of pinewood and fashioned on a lathe, they have two large rounded humps either side of a central depression. You use it by lying on your back on the floor, knees bent so that you can lower yourself on to the roller which is on the floor under the low back. You then lower some of your weight on to the roller and then by moving the body up and down the floor roll the device back and forth under the spine. The two humps of the roller are exactly positioned, either side of the knobs to the spine, to massage the facet joints. The problem ones will be felt as painful when you roll over them. Self-treatment consists of worrying these sore spots by making small excursions back and forth over them. As they become less painful, as they do quite quickly, then you lower more weight on to the roller and so stress the problem joints even more.

Unfortunately, as excellent as these 'Ma Rollers' are, they are very hard to come by. In their stead I have come to rely upon the lowly tennis ball. Not so lowly I suppose, because it must be new and top-quality, and therefore fully tensed with air. It can be used in exactly the same way as the roller. Find the painful spot and lower your back down onto the ball. When you have found the spot, gently wriggle around on the ball so that it hurts. The stiff spinal segment or the stiff facet joint will be unable to move in concert with the others as you roll over the ball. You will not necessarily sense the stiffness, but you will certainly sense the pain. Roll back and forth over the joint a couple of times a day for a minute or two and you will see daily how the pain fades. Always accompany this self-treatment by the appropriate exercises in order to take full advantage of the new freedom it's brought.

I have many patients who are addicted to their tennis ball. Indeed I have even come to the conclusion that no family medical chest is complete without one. If self-treatment is to be taken seriously, this is the best means of self-mobilisation available.

WHAT WILL MANIPULATION ACHIEVE?

Manipulation is particularly useful in unlocking an otherwise mobile healthy joint previously not painful, which has become jammed with an awkward movement.

A physiotherapist will also manipulate a degenerated joint when it is nearly better; when it is just a bit brittle but not really painful. Manipulation at this stage will get the 'spring' back into the joint. This speeds up the later stages of recovery.

There is no doubt that the immediate feeling of 'release' created after a successful manipulation does bring about a feeling of well-being. However, cracking like this is often too rough. Too many tissue fibres are broken so that, although there is that initial sense of freedom, the relief quickly fades. You become addicted to being yanked. Microscopic scar tissue forms around the joint which causes it to become tighter and tighter. The patient feels he needs manipulation more and more frequently to keep himself in the same free state.

As a manipulator myself, I know well the feel of a back which has been manipulated too often. I can feel with my hands that the joints are characteristically over-tough and rubbery. It takes a lot of gentle mobilisation and quite a long time (perhaps months) until the back can be restored to a looser, more comfortable, elastic state.

The other great problem with manipulative treatment, especially if done by a lay manipulator, is that unless the manipulator is a very slick operator indeed it is difficult to accurately localise the manipulation to the required spinal level. All manipulation techniques are done as a gross movement, using the rest of the patient's body for leverage. For this reason it is very difficult to make the vertebral level go that you want to go! Frequently there is a loud crack and everybody is satisfied, but in reality it is the healthy joint above which has been treated and the troublemaker has not been budged.

A more satisfactory approach is to do a lot of preliminary mobilising with the thumbs right in on the spot in order deliberately to prise the vertebra free. Then, when it is moving more freely and one can get a bit more purchase on it, manipulate it.

Manipulation at the culmination of treatment of a problem joint is very necessary for the complete recovery of the joint.

One does not expect the adverse response described earlier because the joint, having been thoroughly worked over during several treatment sessions, is now in a fitter state to accept more aggressive handling.

During the previous mobilisation process, the professional handling of the joint has brought the blood rushing. The state of sluggish inactivity is interrupted by the physiotherapist's thumbs pushing and pulling the vertebrae about. Cleansing, healing blood floods to the site of activity to help the joint cope with the unexpected irritation. Now, with the benefit of an improved blood supply, the tissues revert to a healthier state.

CAN MANIPULATION BE BAD FOR ME?

Manipulation is not dangerous to the healthy individual. It should never be done where there is rheumatoid arthritis, bone cancer or osteoporosis (where the bones become thin and brittle). Here it could be catastrophic.

However, joints should not be over-manipulated. It is easy to tell if you have been too frequently and too aggressively manipulated. Your joints will always have a rubbery, tight, spongy feel and you, the patient, will always be itching to be manipulated anew. It seems these joints give you an almost permanent feeling of being bound up, the only relief being another manipulation. It is another case of 'smoking more and enjoying it less' as you become convinced that you need another quick click to release you.

The joint capsules become scarred and thickened by repeated forceful yanks which have caused microscopic tearing of the tissue fibres. The scarring causes the joint to tighten up even more than it originally was, so the problem snowballs.

As a finale to the course of treatment, we usually manipulate the joint before the patient is finally discharged. We do this to 'clear' the joint. This final demand on the joint ensures that it is fully capable of realising all its freedom and forestalls a recurrence of the problem due to incomplete treatment.

I know exactly what my patients like about these manual therapy techniques. They correspond so closely, it seems, with what they instinctively feel would help their sore backs. Surely, they feel this is how medicine used to be, 'the laying on of hands' so sadly missing in today's impersonal clinical world. The hands, in all their complex simplicity. The benefits are so clear-cut; they can hardly be overstated.

But, like most things in life, effective treatment of backpain is not just a one-sided affair. You as a patient must contribute largely to your own recovery. So far I have outlined my role in easing that painful back. Now I want to tell you about what you can do to help yourself, something you do progressively more of as treatment proceeds.

6

EXERCISE FOR A BACK

PROBLEM

One of the most distressing aspects of a back problem is that the sufferer sees himself as a passive victim of the pain. He feels unable to cope during an attack and equally unable to prevent a recurrence of the problem.

However, you can help yourself. There are one or two things that you can do right in the middle of an attack which will help you get rid of some of that pain (and these will be discussed later). You can also do exercises which directly target the central problem. These exercises help by redressing the structural problems of the jointed skeleton as a whole, problems which by their very existence have made back trouble, sooner or later, an inevitable development. But it must be stressed that these exercises are only indirectly therapeutic. It is not possible to cure a back problem at the outset simply by exercising it. Exercise is of more preventive value than therapeutic value. Its role is always ancillary to specific manual treatment and it should take the form of a specific regime related to your own particular problem rather than indiscriminate general-purpose exercises. Each specific exercise should have a definite aim in view, its role to help in the common purpose of realigning the working skeleton so that the stresses borne by the problem joints are minimised. In this way the problem spots are defused. The exercises are done later on, after treatment has freed you of the acute pain. This is where exercises come into their own. As the back gets less sore, you do more. In effect, you phase in as we the therapists phase out.

However, the benefits derived from general exercise or sport are very different from the benefits of specific exercises. The value of sport is its capacity to rev up the system and put it into a state of full flight, all in the name of good fun. This has the hidden gain of keeping the general musculature toned up, of preventing muscle and ligament contracture and of keeping the joints well oiled and juicy; in short, preventing the skeleton getting out of kilter. Ideally, it prevents back problems starting in the first place.

But the shortcoming of general exercise is that it is not careful enough. It is hardly tailored delicately to undo the bad changes that happen to the joints of the skeleton; more to the point, the blunderbuss effect of sport on the frame, where joints, muscles and tendons are 'railroaded' into participation, often has an unwelcome triggering effect on dormant faulty joints. Invariably sport fails in its task of balancing the joint performance simply because it is not sufficiently balanced or controlled in itself. Too often modern sports are violent and unvarying in their pattern of movement, subjecting the skeleton to fleeting new strains on top of old subtle ones (see 'Sport And The Back' Chapter 7).

Sadly, most of us have skeletons which have a patchy distribution of joints of below-par performance. Some joints are too tight and others are too loose, the result of lack of variety of activity and lack of variety of the postures we use to relax. Always in a chair watching television, hardly moving all evening.

It is then but a small step to 'do something' fairly minor which tips the balance. So often you, the patient, will complain that you hardly did anything to precipitate a particularly nasty bout of backpain. This causes frustration and hopelessness because you feel that if you cannot even sneeze, for example, or pick up the soap from the floor of the shower without disastrous consequences, then how on earth are you going to cope with all the other rigours of life?

But, you see, you really had it coming to you. Your frame was like a car where some of the bolts were rusty, others not screwed up tight enough, yet others were over-tightened so that all 'play' at their union was obliterated. In all, an extremely creaky car. The mechanics of the skeleton can be equally out of balance. And, what is more, this overall poor performance cannot be rectified by attention to just one bolt. Nor can it be rectified by taking the car on a hundred-kilometre run, the equivalent of indiscriminate over-energetic exercising.

It is important, if you want to spend a life as free as possible from aches and pains, that the skeleton is completely balanced in all its physical work. For the skeleton to run harmoniously, there must be a balance of muscle play across all working joints. Smoothly running joint performance can only happen, first, if the joints are not stiff and, second, if the muscles which control movement of the joints are in equally matched working order.

Each muscle group across a joint has an opposite number on the other side of the joint which provides the reciprocal movement for the joint. For example, the biceps bends the elbow and the triceps straightens it again, and vice versa. The opposing group also performs the important, though less obvious, task of controlling the primary movement as it takes place. It does this by slowly relaxing and paying out its length so that the primary movement is controlled, as it were, by the other side. The opposing muscle group keeps its tension and only lets go at a delicately programmed rate so that the primary movement is smooth and purposeful, not jerky and unco-ordinated.

It is important that all paired muscle groups are of equal strength and also of equal length. If the skeleton is bedevilled with joints where the partnered muscle groups are of unequal ability, the joints will chafe. It does not do to have two masters of unequal skill controlling a joint. It leads to grumbling dissent; their threshold is lowered and they are more susceptible to other irritations.

The unwelcome consequence of inequality of strength across a joint is easier to understand than the disturbance caused by inequality of length. If one group is stronger, it will more powerfully pull a joint its own way, more effortlessly than its partner can return it.

Equally so, when it comes to stabilising a joint, as when bracing the back, when both the partners of the pair have to contract statically to hold the joint firm and resist shock, the fact that one group is holding firmer than the other leads to trouble. It would be better if they were both weak rather than one weak and one strong. The simple imbalance causes strain to be tolerated poorly, whereas if they were both weak the resulting joint laxity would help the joint to ride out the storm better. This subtle imbalance of the joint sets up a chronic strain which is the beginning of the joint wearing out.

The stronger a muscle is, the more 'tone' it has. Tone is best described as the tension within a muscle when it is at rest, as if the muscle is in a permanent state of low-grade contraction. The greater the tone, the less extensible the muscle is. This means over a period of time the muscle imperceptibly pulls in its length and becomes shorter. This is bad news for the joint underlying a strong muscle not only because it spends its resting moments being compressed together by the non-relaxing muscle, but also because it is not as stretchy as a weaker muscle and cannot ever let go and release to full stretch. This means that the joint will never enjoy excursions right up to the weaker muscle group's end of range. When it comes to its turn to work the joint, the weaker muscle does not have the power to pull the joint against the resting resistance of the other stronger group. It is therefore harder to work the joint one way than the other. Inequality of movement is set up.

Over a period of time the stronger muscle group adaptively shortens and the weaker muscle group adaptively lengthens and a permanent contracture of the joint comes about.

The elbow is a good example of this problem. If a strong man does more activity where he bends the elbow rather than straightens it, his elbow will start to habitually hang crookedly at the side like that of an ape because he has lost the freedom to straighten out the arm fully.

'Tennis elbow' is a condition caused by inequality in length of paired muscle groups. Because there are many more forehand shots in tennis than backhand, the flexor group on the inside of the forearm which powerfully pulls the wrist through with the racket, gets stronger than the extensor group on the back of the forearm which takes the wrist and racket back the other way in the backhand shot. Because the punchy forehand slash is so powerful, the weaker extensor group on the back of the forearm is at a loss to exert proper control on the movement. They suffer a sudden jerk as they try to steady the wrist, the jerk tugging the muscle where it attaches to the bone at the other side of the elbow.

Furthermore, the strong forehand shot demands such total and instantaneous release of the opposing group that even the shortest delay will also result in the muscle being jarred at the site where the muscle attaches to the bone on the outside of the elbow.

Third, with a backhand shot, because the flexor group is so strong and loath to be stretched out to its full length, it cannot give and pay out freely as the extensors contract to do the shot. This means that as the feeble extensors are pulling the wrist back in the backhand shot the movement is suddenly pulled up short, in full flight, because the strong group has reached the end of its tether. This jars the extensors and again causes a tug to ripple through the muscle and tear the muscle off the bone. This causes inflammation and pain. The familiar tennis elbow pain.

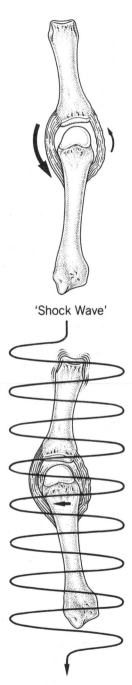

'Shock Wave'

34 Even at rest a joint will suffer strain if held by a pair of muscles of unequal ability. If the joint is shocked, inadequate bracing will cause further damage.

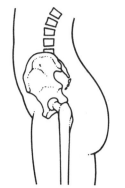

Lordosed lumbar spine

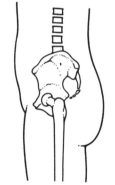

Straight lumbar spine

35.1 Postures of the low back.

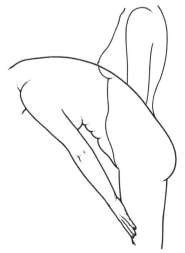

36.1 Pain associated with an increase in the lordotic curve is often relieved by curling forward.

This well-known example of how badly a joint can start to malfunction, producing significantly disabling pain, illustrates only too clearly how important it is in all joints, not least the back, that muscles of balanced ability all work together in harmony to co-ordinate the skeleton.

Thus, you should never concentrate on exercising one muscle group at the expense of all others. The muscles at the front of the spine (the tummy muscles) as well as those behind (the back muscles) and those at the sides of the spine, as well as those at the front of the hips and those at the back of the thigh (the hamstrings), all have to be checked to see if they are equally supple *and* equally strong.

Imbalance of the large skeletal muscle groups which in their ideal efficient state should hold the body in proper postural alignment is the fundamental core of back problems. It takes years to develop. It is not as if you wake up one morning and think: My God, my hip flexors are tight! It will only be obvious to you when you try to assume a correct posture and cannot. Then it will be clear that some muscles are tight and cannot let you go.

Stretching exercises as well as strengthening exercises will make sure that in the future the basic posture of the body is improved thereby forestalling any recurrence.

WHAT EXERCISES SHOULD I DO?

Specific exercises may be necessary to restore parity to coupled muscle groups, but it is no use just exercising indiscriminately.

If you are to take on the job of helping to treat your own back, the parts which you need to stretch or strengthen cannot be understood until the basic differences in posture types are understood. Exercises which are invaluable for one painful back may have a disastrous effect on another.

Backpain is often associated with a posture of the low back which is at variance with the norm. It may be too scooped out and hollow (called a lumbar lordosis) or it may lack any hollow at all, completely flat, or it may even curve the other way (the lumbar kyphosis).

Backpain which is associated with an over-hollow low back usually means that most of the pain is coming from degenerated facet joints. They are grinding under the strain of being rammed down into one another: a subtle impaction effect as the back edges of the vertebrae impinge in a hollowing spine.

Invariably the pain intensifies if you deliberately extend or arch your back, in effect increasing the jamming, but often flexion or bending forward is just as painful because the soft-tissue structures have become accustomed to the spine sitting habitually one way. They have shortened and are disinclined to stretch out the other way.

The single best strengthening exercise for this type of back is to exercise the tummy: *sit-ups.*

Sit-ups should really be called curl-ups because that is what they should be. You must prevent a shearing strain of the low lumbar vertebrae so you 'curl up' rather than 'flip up' to the sitting position. *This must be done with the knees bent*, at first with the feet secured (under the bed or sofa), then feet unsecured as you get better at doing it.

What you are trying to achieve is controlled segmental movement where, like cogs in a wheel, the spine lifts up off the floor one vertebra after the other, to the fully curled position — chin on knees — and down again in the same cat-curling controlled way.

By the way, the real enthusiasts claim that to ensure you get only the tummy muscles working and to eliminate any contribution from the powerful hip flexor muscles you must push your heels into the floor as hard as you can as you sit up. Indeed, it has been found that if the sit-ups are done by flipping up, not by curling, there is even some contribution from the muscles of the back which ideally should remain completely inactive during the exercise. Incidentally, this may account for the increase sometimes observed in backpain after doing poor-quality tummy exercises. Do them better and you will not get pain.

But heels into the floor is too hard for me. Also I fear that the average back sufferer would flail around on the floor like a beetle on its back and get absolutely nowhere. However, do it by all means if you can.

Sit-ups help by building up the strength of the tummy, the retaining wall at the front which straightens the sagging spine. This improves the 'resting posture' of the spine and reduces postural strain. It also means that in its dynamic 'working posture' it is less likely to be strained, whatever work it does. Hence whenever we bend forward, which is the most expansive and generous movement that the spine

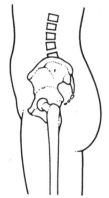

Normal lumbar spine

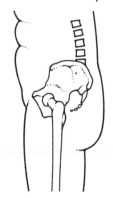

Kyphosed lumbar spine

35.2 Postures of the low back.

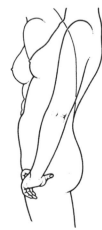

36.2 Pain associated with a lack of normal lumbar curve is often relieved by arching backwards.

has, when the guiding facet joints which control movement are least engaged, that strong retaining wall prevents each little brick-like vertebra from 'shearing' forward off the one below.

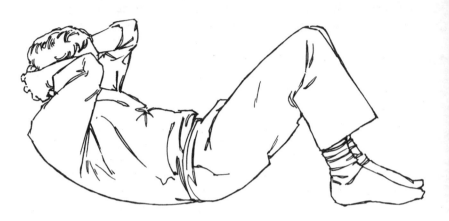

37 Sit-ups should always be done as curl-ups.

Of course the spinal ligaments and natural bony catches of each vertebra which notch the spine together do the bulk of the work holding the spine together, but it is the small, almost incidental movements that will cause you to 'rick' your back, and this is prevented by muscle control.

Curl-ups it is. Remember though that if you do these tummy exercises in the wrong way, you can cause a new and nasty back strain.

It is so common to see sit-ups being done badly. It makes me wince to see the Rugby squad out there on the field all doing their sit-ups and leg-lifts. On the other hand, it makes me think that it won't be long before, one by one, they all file in for treatment. Quality is the clue, not quantity. It is fine segmental control you are trying to achieve, so sit-ups are to be done in a gentle and disciplined way. Up without jerking and grunting and down slowly like rolling out a carpet. Eventually you should easily be able to do thirty sit-ups with hands behind the head and knees crooked and feet unsecured.

Although double leg-lifts, lying flat on your back on the floor and lifting both legs off, are a sort of tummy-strengthening exercise, they are absolutely taboo. Never do them. They create immense back strain by causing the spine to arch perilously with the effort. The arching, brought about by the strong hip muscles pulling on the front of each lumbar vertebra, causes a shearing strain on the lumbar vertebrae which can easily cause trouble. Furthermore this exercise barely strengthens the tummy muscles at all.

There is really only one tummy exercise worth doing and that is the one described. If you have to take time out to do exercises, you might as well make sure they are effective.

The chief architects of perfect curl-ups are the internal and external oblique muscles. These two sheets of muscle wrap around the abdominal wall below the ribs and above the two ear-shaped pelvic bones. The muscle fibres of the external oblique run in an inward and downward direction following the line that fingers take in a pocket while the internal run in a diagonally opposite direction from the base of the rib cage at the front, out and down to the large hip bones. By acting in tandem in contrary directions, these two muscles create a creasing or buckling effect of the front wall of the abdomen. As with all muscle contraction, the fibres shorten in length, bending the torso across its middle to create the perfect sit-up.

This action also causes a significant increase in intra-abdominal pressure, which in turn elongates the lumbar spine within the abdominal cavity. This may explain the therapeutic value of this simple exercise and I can certainly vouch for its efficacy in my own clinics. Pure oblique action involves pelvic rotation as well as creasing at the abdomen. To do this you need to lie on your back on the floor, knees bent in the air. Difficult as it is, attempt to bring the right shoulder and elbow up to touch the left knee. It is an advanced exercise so do not attempt it in the early stages of recovery.

Sit ups done badly are a disaster. In the awkwardness of the effort, the body will do a trick manoeuvre whereby the hip muscles do all the work and the tummy balloons out. The compression effect on the spine is a terrible one. It is rather like creating bend in an unyielding flag-pole by increasing the tension of one of its stays. Eventually the pole bends, but at the expense of imploding it deeper into the ground as the pressure of the stay on the top of the pole increases, bending it over. The hip flexors work like this. They create a compression effect upon the spine and achieve the angulation of the sit-up by pulling the spine forward and bending at the hips. And for most spines, even uncomplaining ones, this is not a good thing to do.

The difference between a good and a bad sit-up is of critical importance. Immense care must be taken to ensure that

38 Pure oblique sit-ups.

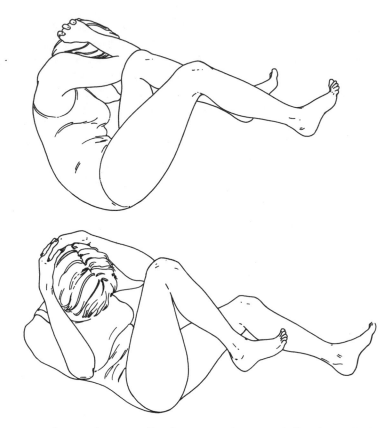

you are doing them well. If you are having difficulties, help yourself up to the sitting position as best you can (without jarring!) and then, once you are in the sitting position, let go of your legs and curl back to the floor. Emphasise a controlled release from the full curl, with your navel sucked in.

If you just cannot do any sit-up at all because of pain, hanging abdominals are an ideal alternative. Mind you, they have their difficulties too, especially for the arms and hands.

Stainless steel chin up bars are available from most sports stores, which you can assemble yourself and attach to a doorjamb at home, following the instructions that come with the kit. Make sure the jamb is solid enough to take your weight and that you wedge the bar in very tightly so that there is no danger of its giving way while you're using it.

Grasp the bar firmly, preferably with gloved hands to prevent blisters, either from the floor if you're tall enough or by stepping off a chair or other object if you're not. Let your legs hang free in mid-air. If the doorway is too low you may have to bend your knees and tuck your feet up behind you. Using the principles of curl rather than flip, slowly but surely bring your thighs from vertical, right up to your chest.

Let me tell you, these exercises are extremely hard work. You will never get your knees up under your chin, but that is the general direction. At first you will only manage two or three lifts and your arms will hurt like mad. But hanging abdominals are valuable. They use the trunk-curling muscles but without spinal compression and shear. There is even some pleasant separation of the lower joints as you hang there — all the benefits of abdominal exercise with a few other advantages thrown in.

If backpain which occurs in conjunction with a flattened lumbar curve is made much worse by bending forward, especially where the movement is interrupted at about twenty degrees by an obvious rolling swivel either to the left or to the right as if 'around' an obstacle, then it is clearly indicative of a low-back problem originating in the disc. Exercises in this instance are aimed at reversing the present posture, that is, increasing the hollowing. The reasons for this are complicated, a matter of minimising the intra-discal pressure. The actual pressure within a disc is at its lowest when we lie flat on the back and at its greatest when we tip forward as we pass through twenty degrees from vertical. The pressure decreases again as we pass right down into the fully curled position, head on knees, when there is a gentle distractive force pulling the vertebrae apart. It also decreases at the extreme of the other movement, extension, as the over-riding of the facet joints at the back of the spine 'lifts' one vertebra off the one below and takes the pressure off the disc.

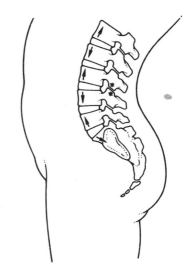

39.1 In extension the impingement of the bony surfaces of the back of the spine takes compression off the disc.

The reason that it is particularly painful to bend at the twenty-degree point is that, unlike a normal healthy disc, a degenerated disc will force a bulge out of the back of the disc space when the pressure within the disc is at its greatest, that is, at the twenty-degree point in the arc of movement as one bends forward.

Unfortunately, as a disc degenerates, the nucleus, that perfect liquid pearl in the centre of the disc, loses its properties to disperse pressure. The nuclear material changes from being fluid in nature to gluey and fibrous. It tracks through the fragmented internal structure of the inner wall of the disc as soon as it is subjected to pressure. Instead of behaving like a strong and resilient rubber ball, the disc behaves more like a perishing rubber ball. It squashes with pressure, and the flaccid walls of the disc distend, particularly with forward bending movements of the spine.

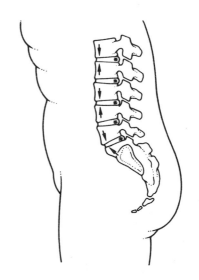

39.2 In flexion facet impingement is disengaged and the posterior walls of the discs balloon with the pinching effect of the front of the discs.

With an acute flare-up of a disc you commonly find yourself fixed just a few degrees short of the twenty-degree mark, unable to go any further ahead because you will maximise peak bulging. But you are just as unable to get back into a more extended position where the pressure within the disc is not so fierce, because the bulge at the back of the disc cannot suck itself in as your torso rolls back over it. By attempting to get back upright, you risk pinching the bulge between the two adjacent margins of the vertebral bodies, and locking it out there. Very painful.

For this type of back there are two valuable exercises. They must both be done lying down so that the intra-discal pressure is at its lowest and the bulge of the disc less.

The first exercise is *passive extension*. This is done lying in the face-down position. At the outset you may even find it a job getting into this position. You may be in a lot of pain and you may need a pillow under the tummy to safeguard your uncomfortable bent shape.

Just lie there and in time you should be able to do away with the pillow and it will be more comfortable to lie flat. Easy to see why we call this exercise passive: you do nothing at all except lie there and let gravity flatten you out straight.

By encouraging extension, we reduce the pressure on the disc by putting the facet joints in a position where they bear more weight, but this also tends to encourage the nucleus to squirt to the other side of the disc and thus reduce the distortion effect on the back wall of the disc.

As you find it easier to get straighter, we then ask you to elevate yourself on to your elbows and stay there for as long as possible and then lower yourself down again to rest. As this in turn gets easier, then push yourself up on the hands so that the arms are straight and the spine is arched backwards. Although this exercise may be quite uncomfortable in the back, if at any stage it creates a worse pain in the leg, then stop and just go back to lying peacefully on the floor on the tummy. If it is too painful to lie on the tummy, then just lie in any position that is comfortable until you are in a less painful state. This may take days (see 'Should I Not Rest in Bed?' Chapter 4).

When you are in a much fitter state and can painlessly push yourself back into extension off the floor, then you should progress the exercise by doing the same manoeuvre in the standing position. Legs planted well apart with the fists thrust into the back of the waist, lean over backwards. Do this several times a day; you cannot overdo it.

This exercise can also be done if you have none of the

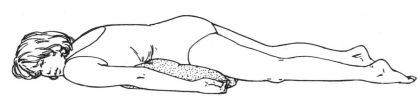

40.1 While you are still bent with pain you will need to lie over pillows stacked under the tummy to get comfortable.

40.2 Slowly and progressively remove pillows until it is comfortable to lie flat.

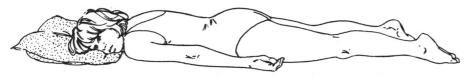

40.3 Then you will stack pillows under the rib-cage to ease your spine gently into an arched position.

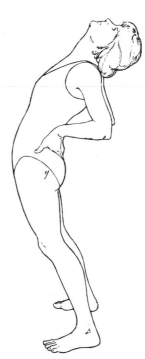

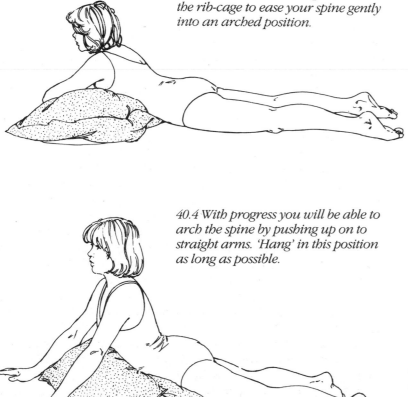

40.4 With progress you will be able to arch the spine by pushing up on to straight arms. 'Hang' in this position as long as possible.

40.5 Eventually, in the standing position, you will be able to do a grand spinal extension, a much needed release for the average spine. This should be avoided if back pain is associated with an increased lumbar lordosis.

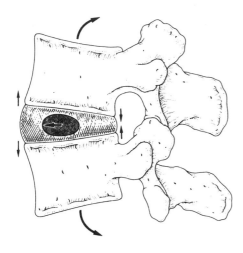

41 In extension the nucleus migrates away from the back wall of the disc.

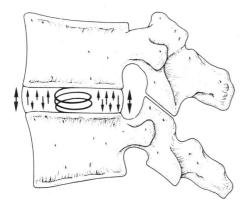

42 The elastic lattice make-up of the disc wall acts like a coiled spring which resists compression.

above drama of a particularly nasty disc problem, but simply have a low back that is habitually too round and lacks the proper hollow. Again this exercise cannot be done too much and will help forestall the type of disc flare-up just described.

As well as encouraging the nucleus of the disc to migrate away from the weak bulging wall, these exercises also simply stretch the spine back on itself and bend it out of its usual crooked shape. This stretch is very valuable to the health of the disc wall as well. The simple reason for this is that the internal structure of the wall of the disc is composed of concentric fibrous rings, coiled in alternating opposite directions like high-tensile springs. With each successive layer in the wall (the annulus), of which there are many, the fibres of each lattice layer are arranged at right angles to one another. This results in a continuous lattice of springs which have the invaluable effect of countering the heavy compressive weight of torso above by thrusting the vertebrae apart (see diagrams 41 and 42).

When the spine has been immobilised for a long time through pain, the soft tissues that clothe the spine adaptively shorten. These soft tissues exert a suffocating tethering effect on the spine and keep it permanently clamped together, disabling the spring effect.

Stretching the walls out again, freeing them from the restrictive soft-tissue binding, liberates the spring properties of the disc. The whole encircling wall of the disc needs to be stretched, including the troublesome back wall, and this is where the *passive flexion* comes in. But beware!

As I said earlier, this is the most risky of all exercises for a discogenic problem, but that does not mean that you shy away from it and never attempt it. Take great care and take your time, but if you are too nervous do not try it. The anxiety will tighten you up and thwart the aim. But just remember that you should be able to do all things, and to give up at the start is defeat at the outset with little likelihood of ever getting any better. If in doubt, don't. But do bear in mind you are trying to get cured and you will *not* be until you can do all movements of the spine normally and automatically.

Initially the flexion must be done lying down so that the pressure within the disc is at a minimum. Lie comfortably on your back on your bed. Gather up one leg behind the knee with both hands and gently pull the knee to the chest and gently bounce it there. Progress the exercise by bouncing the knee harder as the pain abates and then gather both knees to the chest and bounce them both.

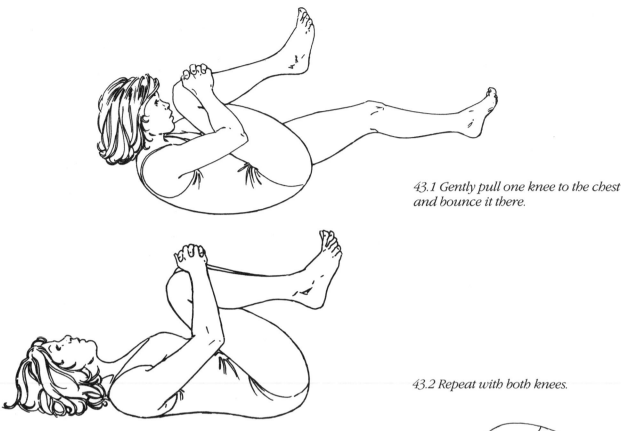

43.1 *Gently pull one knee to the chest and bounce it there.*

43.2 *Repeat with both knees.*

This exercise is progressed further by flexing the spine in the standing position, that is, by bending forward. It is normal to feel hesitant about bending forward when the back hurts, especially this sharp stabbing hurt as you pass through the painful arch of movement, but it is imperative that you *do* bend. You may need to start off initially by lowering yourself around the bulge by crawling down the legs with the hands on the thighs (see 'Is Bending Bad for Me?' Chapter 8).

The important thing, though, is to do the full bend, because that is where all the benefit is. Lower yourself into the full bend and hang there bouncing. It becomes quite relaxing after a while.

The next aspect of this chapter on exercise deals with joints in the near vicinity of the low back which by their abnormal function may also prevent the low back from returning to its former problem-free state. The muscles and ligaments of the hips have the greatest role to play in this respect.

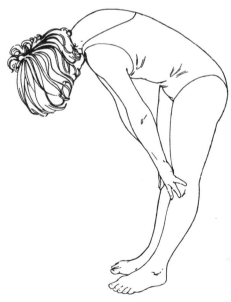

44.1 *When you feel loath to bend, help yourself by climbing down your legs.*

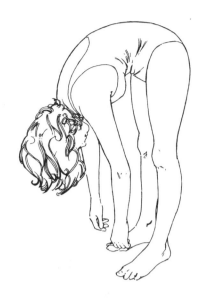

44.2 When you have arrived at the fully flopped position, relax and bounce.

In the case of a lordotic lumbar spine, it is common that the hip flexors are tight as are the low back extensors. At the same time the tummy muscles are weak as are the muscles of the buttocks.

To stretch the hip flexors, lie on the back on the bed or preferably on a firm table and let the leg hang off the side edge of the bed, so that the hip falls back. Then, holding behind the knee, pull the other leg up on to the chest, without allowing the other leg to come up as well. Bounce it there. Repeat the same procedure with the other leg. As the hip flexors get more stretched out, perhaps you could ask your partner to exert pressure on the thigh of the straight leg to increase the stretch (see diagram 45).

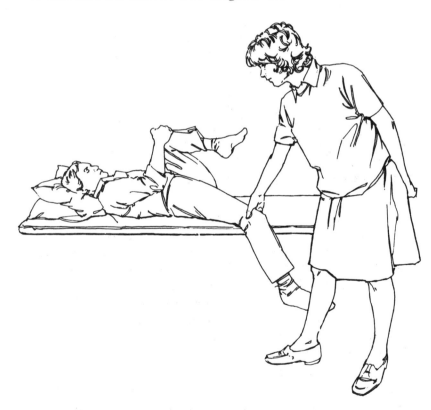

45 The hip-flexor stretch for the right leg.

The way to stretch out the tight low-back muscles is to lie on the back and roll up into a ball. Do this by holding on to both thighs behind the knees, if necessary linking the forearms. In this position, pull the thighs up closer to the chest so that you feel a stretching sensation in the low back. Do not be afraid to feel this pain; it is only beneficial (see diagram 46).

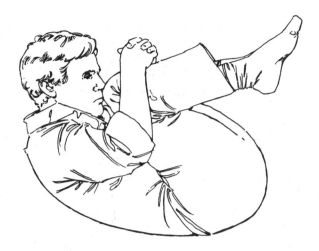

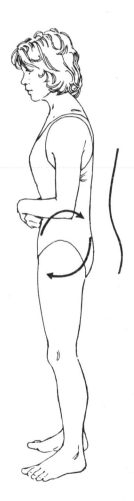

Another exercise which should frequently be done involves statically pulling the tummy in and nipping the bottom in, which swivels the pelvis around so that the de-rotation of the pelvis takes out the hollow of the low back.

Make sure that the shoulders do not droop. Think about it all the time because it is your basic posture that you are trying to change. With the help of the new added strength of the muscles that count, as well as the new added freedom of muscles which formerly would not let go, you will find it easier and easier to find and hold this more satisfactory posture (see diagram 47).

The exercises for those backs which sit habitually in a position of reversed lumbar lordosis, or a flat back, are as follows (see diagram 48).

Lie face down on the floor, not on the bed, and lift the head and shoulders up off the floor in a back-arching movement. This is quite easy to do and should be progressed fairly quickly to incorporate the legs in the lift, too. When that is achieved fairly comfortably you should also incorporate the arms in the backward-arching posture, stretched out above the head. Thirty is the optimum number.

Spines that sit and stand in a permanent slumped position make you, the sufferer, very tired. This is because the spine does not stay upright effortlessly and requires constant muscle action to keep it vertical. However, you will find that the exercise quite rapidly gets easier and that you will quickly benefit from the reduced postural strain.

The long spinal muscles running up the back with their new-found strength easily succeed in reducing the tiring mechanical leverage brought about by the heavy upper body

47 Humping the low back by nipping the buttocks under and rolling the pelvis back.

125

being carried in front of the centre of gravity. They pull the head and torso back into a less stressful position, aligned properly along the line of gravity. Thereafter the back sits stacked happily balanced upon itself, well supported from below by the spine arching gracefully down in its natural spinal curve. That tired aching disappears.

The most important mobilising exercise for a flat or slumped lumbar spine is a passive sustained stretch lying face down on the floor with pillows stacked up under the ribcage. This gently forces the spine around into an unaccustomed hollow. You have to stay there for several minutes a day. When the going gets easier and it is a breeze you should progress the exercise to pushing up on extended arms so that you are forcing the spine even further back. Eventually it should be done while standing by thrusting both hands in hard on either buttock and bending over backwards.

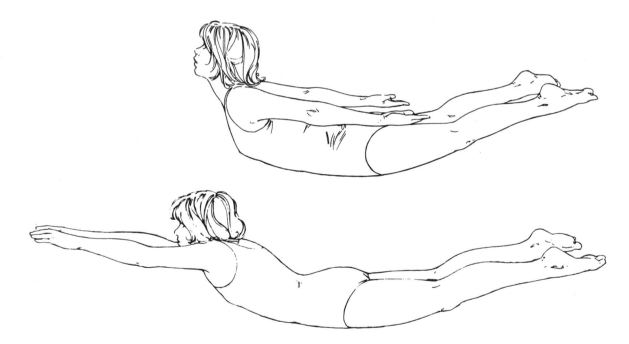

48 The back-arch can be done with the hands beside the body initially, but then progress to hands stretched above the head.

As another measure, it is often useful and very relaxing to lie prone in bed for a while before you go to sleep. The whole skeleton loves this welcome change from a day spent hunched over in studied concentration. It is a step towards redressing the imbalance.

Note, however, that you should not lie in this position without a pillow under the tummy if you are of the other postural type with the back too hollow (see 'In Which Position Should I Sleep?' Chapter 9).

This exercise is invaluable but it is not important for actually stretching the muscles of the tummy. Although these are commonly weak, they are rarely tight. Rather, it is aimed at stretching the soft tissue structures that clothe the front of the spine itself which by their tightness keep it perpetually bowed over.

Another stretching exercise for releasing the fixed abnormal posture of the flat back is the hamstring stretch. When they are tight, these muscles, which attach to the back of the pelvis, keep it rotated in a backward direction and roll the spine into a hump.

The least stressful way to start this exercise is to lie on the back on the floor and, holding on to the action leg behind the knee, bend the leg towards the chest. From this position straighten the leg by pushing the heel up into the air. It is important to lead with the heel; as it is also important to stop the pelvis of the other side rolling back as the tension increases in the muscle.

When you have achieved a fair degree of stretch, which takes a week or so, doing a few minutes twice a day, then the exercise is to be progressed by performing it standing up. Find a low surface such as a stool, about forty-five centimetres off the floor. Support the heel of the action leg on the stool, and with the leg straight bend the head down towards the knee. Do not allow the knee to flex and do not allow the pelvis to twist away from the action leg. Do these stretches several times a day for a couple of minutes and be sure to progress it by raising the level of the support as soon as the tightness abates (see diagrams 50 and 51).

There is one instance where strengthening the spine itself is of value. This is where a segmental joint in the spine has become loose or weak — the 'unstable joint'. This type of back, with a weak link in the middle, is like a broken reed. It keeps folding up under pressure or when caught by an unguarded movement. In this case it is important to strengthen that link and bind it back together strongly with good strong muscles.

Another familiar feature of a spine which harbours a weak link is the typical way one gets up from the bent-forward position. You find it impossible to get yourself up and feel you must climb up the thighs with the hands to get back to vertical. Equally typical is the feeling that the back is going to give way and collapse if you attempt to bend forward a few

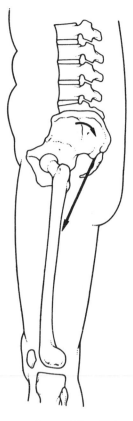

49 Short hamstrings will pull the pelvis around so that the spine bumps.

degrees. Most common is an inability to bend over the washbasin in the morning because the back feels it will give way or go into a painful spasm.

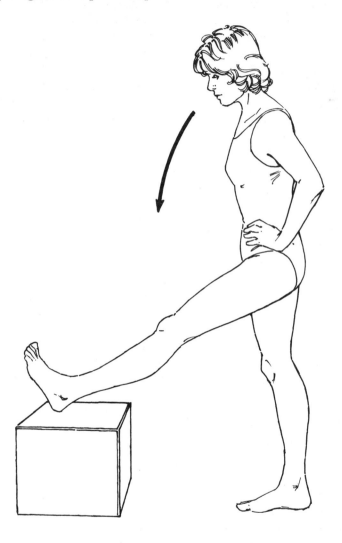

50 The first phase of a hamstring stretch of the left leg. Attempt to bring the nose towards the knee.

As an intuitive protective reflex, the sufferer attempts to reduce the shearing strain across the loose lumbar vertebra during the recovery movement by tucking the bottom forward under the spine so that he is placing the lower joints directly under the overhanging spine above. The centre of gravity is moved forward and recovery is made easier. This phenomenon is called 'reversed lumbar/pelvic rhythm' and is in fact used as a treatment technique to initiate the spine again in the art of bending. This particularly applies to those spines that have not dared to bend for years, where the sufferer feels apprehensive in the extreme about even contemplating such a manoeuvre. As we shall see later, it is imperative that the spine does bend, no matter how insecure it feels.

It is always preferable, when starting to bend the spine again, to do the bend in reverse. This means lowering yourself down the legs with the hands on the thighs to the fully flopped-forward position, and then rising, using the efforts of the back alone without help from the hands. The routine to bear in mind when trying to get up from the fully stooped position is as follows: you must contract the muscles of the tummy and the buttocks together to roll the pelvis back to initiate the movement. After tucking the buttocks under, as a secondary action the spine comes up. By bracing the tummy and tightening the buttocks we unfurl up to vertical.

The 'long' back muscles, which are the obvious ones we feel as two strong ropy cords down either side of the spine, have no ability to hold the individual spinal segments in place. In fact they will do the reverse. They act rather like

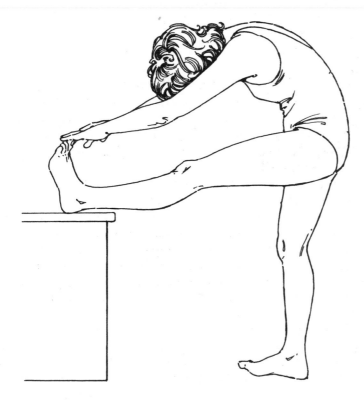

51 A progression of the same manoeuvre using a higher supporting surface.

129

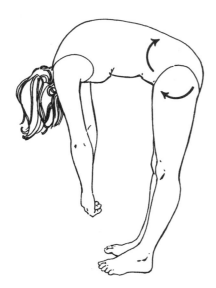

52.1 The action of 'unfurling' to vertical from the fully flopped position is initiated by tucking the bottom under and rolling the pelvis back.

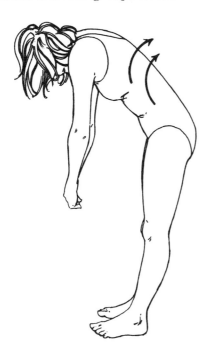

52.2 After the pelvis has fully rolled back, the spine uncurls to vertical.

the stays of a flagpole. They keep us upright once we are upright. They keep the spine erect against gravity, but they have no control over the individual segments between. This is the job of the small 'intrinsic' spinal muscles which pass from one vertebra to the next and keep the spine snugly intact. They make sure that each vertebra sits securely on the one below and does not slip forwards or backwards.

However, it has been shown that when the long back muscles are in spasm, which happens as a matter of course whenever the back is in a state of alarm because of pain, the over-action of the large strap-like muscle running down the back causes an automatic reflex inhibition of activity of the delicate muscles which have the job of controlling the integral fine movement of all the intervertebral segments. The bulky 'macro' muscles contract in one clumsy and permanent contraction and create a bowstring effect on the spine. Conversely, the 'micro' muscles which master the intricate composite movements become paralysed into inactivity and the intrinsic stability of the spine is greatly threatened.

If there is spasm — and you will always know because the back will feel unnaturally hard and stiff — the best way to get rid of it is gently to stretch it. The same applies with any muscle in cramp, be it in your back or in your calf in bed at night: gently elongate the muscle fibres which have contracted in their length.

The way to do this for the back is again to lie on the back and gently, one leg at a time, bring the knee, by holding behind the knee, up on to the chest. When it is there, gently bounce it. Then do the other one. As the spasm subsides, then do both together, but do not try to do this too soon. The combined weight of both legs is unwieldy and may threaten the peacefulness of the exercise.

So the intrinsic muscles have the invaluable role of stabilising the individual spinal segments which go to make up the spine. However, this is a subtle role and the degree of contraction of the individual small muscles is not great. We have found that the same muscles are at their most active when bringing the spine from fully curled position to upright. Once the spine is upright in its erect, relatively stable position, then the long back extensors take over and hold it there.

Therefore, the way to strengthen these muscles is to make them do that movement. Lie face down off the edge of a secure table so that from the hips upward you are suspended in mid-air but head hanging down to the floor, with someone holding on to your legs. From that position you slowly uncurl, from the base of the spine upwards, so that the head comes up last. Once again (as with the abdominal exercises) the emphasis is on individual segmental movement of the spine where one vertebra after the other comes up in a controlled unfurling movement. The emphasis again is on quality not on quantity. Thirty is the optimum number.

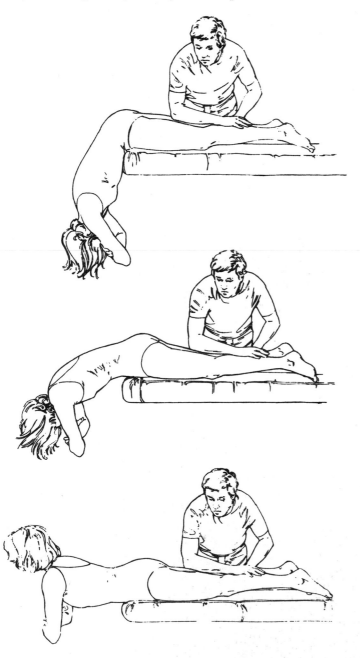

53.1 To improve the intrinsic strength of the spine, hang off the end of a high bench or table with the legs secured.

53.2 53.3 By sucking in the stomach and rolling the pelvis back, unfurl from the fully dropped-down position up to the horizontal.

131

A universal 'best-seller' exercise which is effective at helping just about every spinal problem is the spinal rolling exercise. It is also done lying on your back. Gather both knees up on to your chest and hug them there. In that position gently rock backwards and forwards along the length of the spine. The stiff link will be painful as you roll over it. That is the part that you should be concentrating on, worrying it as you roll back and forth over it (see diagram 54).

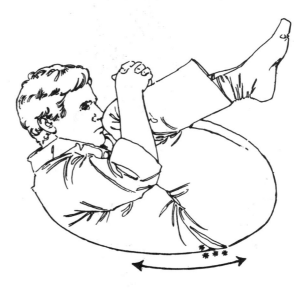

54 The best self-mobilisation technique is to roll the weight of the body back and forth over the problem link.

The value of this exercise is that it passively mobilises each vertebra as you roll your weight over it. In turn each bone glides forward. It should be done in a completely relaxed way so that if you can keep the momentum going it has a mesmerising and comforting effect.

If you are trying to localise the action to improve the functioning of L.4 or L.5, the two lowest vertebrae, you may need to straighten out your legs a bit more to bring the centre of gravity further down the spine to where the problem is. The amplitude of the movement should be very small, otherwise you will spend too much time rolling over all the healthy vertebrae and not getting anything done.

As normality returns, more vigorous exercises such as toe-touching from a standing position can be started. Again, thirty bounces to the floor is about the right number.

7

SPORT AND THE BACK

Today's world is sport mad. We are all led to believe that with a bit more exercise we would all be superhuman. Countless people say to me: 'But why, when I play all this sport, do I still have a bad back?' It is a myth that all sport is actually good for you. It might be good for your head but it may have given you your bad back.

Sport is good for heart and lung function. Blood races through the system; sweat pours out and rids the body of impurities; the lungs are exercised, filling up and emptying of good clean air. But, as a general rule, sport, particularly the more physical and aggressive types, is positively bad for the skeleton. It is a hard grind for the joints.

The prime value of sport is *stretch*. The sports which are valuable are those which do not decree monotonous stereotyped movements (tennis, golf) but those which encourage spontaneous uninhibited movement of unlimited variety; the more generous and willowy the better, the less contrived the better.

Soccer is better than ballet, if you call ballet a sport, because its spontaneous reflex agility compared to the studied precision of ballet, makes for an emancipated skeleton. Ballerinas suffer quite bad backs for just this reason. The range of movements incorporated in their balletic repertoire is admirable, but because the beauty of the art derives from fine precision and graceful control all natural actions of the joints are excessively monitored to eliminate the possibility of any unplanned movements creeping in. Thus, the benefit of going to the end of movement range is denied the joints because there is not enough jaunty 'romp' in the movement to elasticate the joints; not enough flashes of free movement to trounce blood through the joints and keep them fresh and young. All work, no fun.

On the other hand, it is very bad for joints to have no exercise at all. They will quickly tighten up and dry out. With total inactivity the bones themselves de-mineralise and become brittle. Therefore, you can see that a bad arrangement is one of moderate inactivity followed by bone-crunching sport. A stretching sport is fine, but not a bone-cruncher. The worst I can think of, which harbours this combination of brutal non-stretch following inactivity is sky diving, or parachute jumping. There they all sit, hunched up and cold, waiting for their aircraft to reach a high enough altitude. Then they all pile out of the door, free-fall for a bit and then land — crunch — through two legs, strong though they might be, which cannot hope to absorb such a shock. A hard and heavy thud as the spine telescopes up into itself.

Lots of sports are very unnatural. Think about the awkward contortions of a hurdler, for example, bunching up and twisting over the gate, thumping down hard on the leading leg and then pulling the rest of the body over while taking weight on that leg.

It sounds as if I don't like sports. It's not true. Table tennis is excellent. It is quick and light. The playing area is small so that there is a minimum of long run-ups with hefty thumping down on the floor. There are multifarious ways to swing and hit the ball involving as much stretch as you like. The bat is small and light and does not create unfavourable leverage as it is wielded through the air. And, lastly, it is extremely energetic. In no time the players work up a good sweat.

The sad truth of the matter is that so many sports over-use and abuse the joints. Too often they require strength rather than stretch, and strength invariably within repetitive patterns of movement. Sport, the modern mode of outlet for stifled anxiety and spluttered spleen, channels all its power through a few regimented avenues of release. It is against the rules to deviate from the given way.

Such repetitive and aggressive joint activity, back and forth within unvarying confines, wears out the joints. Stereotyped movements do not take the joints on excursions into enough areas of joint freedom and they over-trammel the limited territory which they do use. The harder you play a sport, the more trouble you will store up for yourself.

The last item of bad news about sport is that, even if the sport does serve the requirements of adequate stretch with only a modicum of repetitive stuff, it still may not possess the qualities that will cure you of a back problem. Although it may involve a lot of the sort of generous flourishing movement fit to keep any spine trim and elastic, it is unlikely to be able to zero in on and activate a particular stiff link and loosen it.

Sporting movement is not sufficiently careful to be therapeutic. It is unlikely to bring about the right movement at the right time, the right degree of push in the right direction. It usually either bypasses the joint by allowing the neighbouring joints to do the work or it forces a stiff joint too far and hurts it. Sometimes, if a soft-tissue injury is in its final stages of recovery it will be finally cured by going out for a long run or playing a gentle game of tennis, but if it is not quite ready it will provoke the problem anew and add to your troubles.

YOGA

Yoga is as clever as they come. It originated as long ago as 600 B.C. and today exists as a brilliant discipline of exeptional physical and mental subtlety. It is a collection of postures demanding stretch, balance and strength. But its focus on breathing makes it a gently calming and centring process which sets it apart from so many other forms of physical training today.

The inherited flaw in the human skeleton is that with time, it tightens at the joints. The reason for this is two-fold. Firstly, tissues lose juice with age and secondly, we use our joints without imagination. Not only do we repeat the same movements over and over but most of the useful movements take place within a meagre range of the joints' available freedom. This means that after a period of time our skeletons all show the same pattern of mobility loss. We become like puppets with some of the strings pulled too tight. But in all of us, the same strings are the tight strings and we all fall victim to the same complaints. Where yoga helps is that it recognises the complicated way that joints tighten and it reverses the pattern. Take the shoulder for instance. The first movement it will lose as it gets older is the ability for the arm to go above the head. But that restriction will always co-exist with others which you might not be so aware of. In the shoulder's case, an outward twisting action of the arm in the socket as it goes up.

What I am saying is that each 'functional' movement is made up of a composite of many 'accessory' movements and it is these movements, as integral components of the over-all movement which yoga targets. A yoga arm-stretch for instance, will always incorporate this hidden outward rotation movement of the arm. A composite stretch incorporating accessory stretches, will be much more effective than a simple stretch. Or, put another way, in a stretching regime, the quickest way to regain overall movement is a composite stretch rather than a simple. In this way, yoga is much more sophisticated than the average aerobics or calisthenics workout. The yoga postures are beautifully designed to target many co-existing patterns of stiffness in the one stretch. It also works on several joints at the one time. What is more, it highlights certain key problem spots, (like the shoulders and the hips) which by their existence alone are the very cornerstones of a very much more widespread problem.

So yoga targets incipient kinks in the skeleton and by re-establishing background or accessory movement in all of our joints, it coaxes us around to normal.

Yoga also enhances high-performance coordination. This it does by facilitating 'fine joint play'. Anyone employing so-called high performance motor activity of his skeleton, must have joints which can do what he wants them to do. In the case of the delicate work of the brain surgeon or the golfer sinking a hole-in-one, the coordinated effort of the muscles and the joints is remarkable. To achieve absolute accuracy, the muscles need to constantly make fine adjustments in the joints' angle of action. But they can only 'line the joints up' optimally if the joints are slack enough to accomodate this sort of internal manoeuvering. The looser the joints are, the more able they are to shuffle and adjust and the more precise will be their ultimate performance. One reason for physical clumsiness is imperfect joint positioning. As we line up, poised in space to throw a dart or thread a needle, we do a good job if all our joints do a good job. Yoga keeps us in that optimal state of loosely active preparedness and in getting us there what is more, it winds back the clock and keeps our joints young.

So, yoga can not only make a super performer out of you by fine tuning physical skills which you already have, it can also stop a lesser achiever sliding backwards. It is preventative. It can stop you silently slipping into crotchetiness. It slows your deterioration. Furthermore, if you have lapsed and you need attention, it is infinitely therapeutic. There is an enormous variety of postures from which to choose, from the very gentle to the immensely demanding. I advise supervision until you are well initiated and then you can do things on your own at home. I warn you! Get prepared to be seduced.

JOGGING

Running and its milder version, jogging, are a great release but they do more for the mind than for the body.

Those who jog — and I am one of them — feel an almost irresistible need to get out and burn off some energy, particularly after hours spent labouring over a desk or stitched up with anxieties and frustrations. Running does have a calming effect. It puts you in a frame of mind where automatically all worries assume more normal proportions. Solutions to problems become clearer.

This can only help the spine because stress can have an adverse physical effect if left unchecked. With stress, the skeleton starts to crack up. At rest the muscles never quite relax and as a result, when you do have something purposeful to do with those muscles, they tire more easily. Muscle strains happen far more readily.

The joints, too, suffer because they are kept cramped up under tight muscles. Their nutrition is reduced because the changes of pressure within the joint, corresponding to periods of strong physical work followed by periods of complete lay-off, are less marked. Instead of the blood supply flooding through the joint as it does in the floppy respite following activity, the blood has to be squeezed through the permanently tense tissues.

Strenuous physical exertion 'washes out' stress. All energy reserves are called in and it seems that energy that was being spent on anxiety is converted into physical energy. Thereafter, it seems easier to relax, unwind and lead a more ordered life.

Jogging is one of the best ways to achieve release of pent-up angst. The element of spontaneity is a valuable one. When you feel like letting rip you can; you do not have to get a team together or hire a court or wait until the weather improves. You can also do it wherever you are, on the beach, in the mountains, on holiday, at work at lunchtime. But, most important of all, you can do it at your own pace.

However, benefits apart, it must be said that jogging is detrimental to the joints. It really bashes them around. Unlike walking, especially long, light loping-stride walking, where all the joints glide freely with a minimum of jarring, jogging greatly increases the stresses on joints by piling on the pressure of weight through the joint.

It helps if you run in a way that increases the mobility of the hips and the ankles. This will not only spare them excess trauma when running but will also maximally save the spine by keeping them in a better condition to protect it. The more elastic the hips, the better able they are to absorb shock before it travels up to the spine. For this reason it is imperative to run with as long a stride as possible. This fully extends the hips and opens them out.

It is important to note that when hips develop osteoarthritis, when the function of hip joints starts to deteriorate, simply as a consequence of our getting on in years, the first movement that starts to reduce is this backward or extension movement. Running with long strides helps to keep the hips young by preserving this extension movement.

There is a lot of debate over whether one should land on the heels or on the toes. There is absolutely no doubt that running on the toes greatly minimises jarring shock which reverberates up to the spine. As the foot falls on the ground and the 'super-weight' of the body descends down on to it, the muscles of the calf contract so that the weight is lowered slowly to the ground rather than thudding down hard with no break to the fall.

This makes a lot of work for the calf muscles and their tendon, the Achilles tendon, which is all very well if they are not causing you trouble. However, if you are having Achilles trouble, then my only advice is to make the descent as minimal as possible. The higher you leap into the air, the further you have to come down and the harder the crash. If you creep along so that the feet barely clear the ground, even though you will be landing on the heels, you will be sparing the spine.

A smooth grassy surface is the best thing of all for the jogger: the smoother the better, because bumps and potholes represent an obvious danger of jarring.

The rubberised tracks of athletics grounds are also good to run on. Not only do they sink as the foot strikes the ground, but they also spring back as the weight leaves the surface and propel the body forward.

Whatever the surface you run on, all jogging is greatly influenced by the type of footwear you use. Today there is an infinite variety of jogging shoes to be bought. The best are those which are light in weight and those which have the thickest and the spongiest soles, especially under the heel. Never jog in the old-fashioned plimsolls with their paper-thin rubber soles. The greater the shock-absorption qualities of the sole, the better the shoe.

However, having said all this, it would be negligent of me not to dwell a little longer on the negative effects of running.

Some of my most difficult encounters as a therapist have been breaking the bad news about running. For some, the spectre of life without running brings on a kind of caged-animal hysteria. I do hate being the bearer of bad tidings but I have to make them realise the very real dangers lie ahead.

It is only now that we are seeing joggers or runners twenty years down the track, so to speak. Their skeletons are often appallingly gnarled, with trouble developing at all the major weight-bearing joints. Their intellectual capacities are in peak working order, but you should see their bodies! They have to recognise that there *are* other sports which can bring the same benefits without the damage. It is often a wife who sees the warning signs. She will relate how her husband gets out of bed and 'creeps around like an old man' until he has a shower and gets moving. Of course, he rarely listens to his wife and goes blithely on . . . until he ends up seeing some-one like me!

As has been said before, it is the combination of a seden-tary working life and aggressive endurance running, usually on hard surfaces, that causes all the mischief — going from one extreme to the other with never so much as a hint of a warm up or a stretch beforehand. In the last few years I have become a lot tougher with runners. I no longer beat about the bush with them. If they accept my formula then I will continue to see them, but the conditions are strict. A half hour of stretch, preferably yoga beforehand, sixty curl-ups before and thirty curl-ups after and toe touches at every traffic light, briskly up and down for as long as you're stopped.

AEROBICS

Aerobics is on the right track as an activity for the back, but it is a bit violent. It is commonly taken up by the unfit in a frantic attempt suddenly to get fit. In one quick session people demand all sorts of things of the body which it has not done for years, probably since childhood. But the skele-ton is not fit. It is not the well-oiled, freely functioning ma-chine that it might be and it readily registers strain.

However, aerobics is so much more useful than, say, the gyms where the emphasis is on strength, strength and more strength. The difference is very important. Aerobics involves a very good variety of stretch. In a good class, all the joints are targeted, one after the other, and the habitually tight ones, common to us all, are worked harder than the less troublesome ones.

The main risk with these classes is 'too much too soon'. Many of the exercises are so physically demanding, both the stretches and the strengthening ones, that there is quite a high risk of causing a variety of strains, especially in the early stages. Success depends on carefully stepping up the level of difficulty and endurance of the exercises. If you get there without straining yourself, then you will be very fit indeed. It is a good way to keep fit once you are fit but not an ideal way of getting there.

The whole point about aerobics with all that frenetic exercising and running on the spot is to increase the rate of oxygen uptake of the body. As this increases, the level of fitness increases. For this reason it is absolutely imperative that the workout is done in a room or auditorium where there is lots of fresh air. It is very common and entirely counter-productive to swelter away in a room where there is not a single window that opens or an air-conditioning unit that works. It is not uncommon for everybody to stagger out feeling worse rather than better after one of these sessions.

SWIMMING

Unlike many, I am not such a great fan of swimming. I find it such a nuisance getting to a pool, undressing, swimming, showering, dressing, drying hair, etc. The overall benefit is hardly worth the effort. A few specific exercises you can do at home are just as beneficial.

Swimming can even be bad for you if you complain of a backache which is made much worse by arching backwards, almost invariably associated with a spine which has an increased lumbar lordosis. Swimming on the front has the undesirable effect of allowing the back to sag, which immediately creates pain in the back. Those people who can barely drag themselves out of the pool because the back is so painful obviously have this problem. In the prone swimming position, the lower lumbar facet joints at the back of the spine close up. If the joints are irritable in any way, swimming freestyle or breast stroke will immediately make matters worse.

On the other hand, lumbar disc problems at any level benefit from swimming face down. They are comfortable in this position because they enjoy almost any activity which extends the spine. These problems will always feel better with the breast stroke and freestyle because the extension of the spine reduces the intra-discal pressure. However, any position in the water will be a comfort to a problem disc because the reduction of weight greatly reduces the pressure within the disc.

Ploughing forty times up and down a pool, pushing a bow-wave along in front of you and churning the surface of the water into a seething froth of foam does not do any back a great deal of good. It is the free and generous movement with the body buoyed up by the water which brings about all the benefit. The reduction in weight makes it easy to move fully and effortlessly, thus exercising the joints.

The best thing to do in a pool is the typical hydrotherapy routine, hanging on to the rail that runs around the side at water-level height with your back to the wall. In this position do all sorts of free trunk movements with the knees drawn up to the chest. Do not do any straight leg-kicks because you run the risk of straining the spine.

When you do swim, then make it as gentle and rhythmic as possible, without straining.

TENNIS

Like lots of sports, tennis fails to bring to the skeleton a limitless variety of movement. It consists of a series of hard smashes, all within the same few patterns of movement, using the same lot of muscles over and over again. Like all repetitive sports, especially those which encourage fierce competition, even aggression, tennis traps the player in an exercise groove. In fact he will even play a bad shot if he allows a lapse in concentration to let him deviate to the slightest degree from the set movement format.

Once again, tennis may be exhilarating because it is undeniably a pleasant game but it will not provide benefit, because its movements are so stereotyped. It does not liberate the skeleton. The same batch of muscles are constantly being called in, over and over again.

As I have said several times so far in this book, general healthiness of joints is dependent on those joints having universal freedom to move fully in any direction they have the potential to go in. If they show a limitation to go in any direction, it will not be long before they start being painful. Tennis has this major drawback.

Sports which are very useful are those which encourage the skeleton to move itself in every way. The best sports are non-contact ball sports such as netball, basketball, soccer, table tennis. All of these provide a lot of variety of movement and a lot of stretch. Stretch is the all-important factor. Before a game of tennis it is advisable to stretch the body, easing the joints out of their kinked constrictions. This balances the pull of muscles across the joints, and makes for greatly improved co-ordination during the game.

Lack of consistency of output of energy, especially in doubles, also makes for back trouble. Activity alternates between leisurely standing-about phases and sudden explosive bursts, all the time waving a heavy racket in the air. There you are standing in the middle of the court thinking that no ball can get past you, when one comes lobbing over the net, just a little too short for comfort. You spring into action to make a lurch at the ball — Bang! The back goes.

Trim, taut and terrific players who have better co-ordination are less likely to wrench their joints than the fair-weather player.

The racket is also a bit of a problem. Its length and weight create a long lever which throws a great strain on the spine, especially at full stretch, though this is more likely to affect the shoulder and neck part of the spine.

Tennis also involves a lot of thumping down on a hard court surface which judders the spine. The softer the surface (ideally grass) the better. Clay courts are hard but at least they have the advantage that they allow the players to slide a bit as the foot hits the ground, thus taking a lot of the shock out of landing.

However, any adverse effects of tennis can be partially minimised by having good strong tummy muscles (sit-ups again) and bouncy cushioning tennis shoes, both of which greatly reduce jarring shock either when landing heavily or lunging at some runaway ball.

In defence of tennis, it is, spinally speaking, a better sport than squash. Squash involves a lot of quick and unplanned contorted movements. Tennis is at least a safer version of racquet-and-ball sport if your back is troubling you but you feel you must play something.

GOLF

Golf, unfortunately, is a one-sided activity. It repeatedly wrenches the spine one way as you take a swipe at the ball. Joints are healthy when they have a multi-directional freedom. Golf does not encourage this. In fact, I cannot think of another sport offering less variety of movement. Tennis at least has forehand and backhand strokes and a nice throw into a full extension with the service. Golf movements are completely monotonous.

All that standing about waiting for the other fellow to hit his ball isn't too beneficial either. The old tummy starts to sag. Indeed, as the spine settles into a deeper lumbar curve it may become more and more difficult to bend over to get the ball; or, alternatively, the back may feel fine while you are playing but when it comes to getting into the car afterwards you can hardly bend to do so.

The fact that the spine becomes cast by so much standing around also means that the frequent bends to the ground to pick up the ball are often done as a bad bend rather than as a good one. So often we see it done like a geriatric granny with the legs planted wide apart, the huge abdomen lowered down between the thighs and the stiff arched spine tipped forward by bending at the hips. The shearing strain induced on the low lumbar joints is enormous and one often sees the protective hand fly unconsciously to the back to brace it for the inevitable stab of pain. The bend would be so much more beneficial, not to mention painless, if it were undertaken with a proper curling motion of the spine, helped by a restraining hand to help brace the tummy.

Strong tummy muscles are a must for golfers. They will prevent the forward sag of the spine while standing and they will protect the spine from shearing strain as you do your various bends down to pick up the ball.

It is not uncommon to start feeling stiff on your way around the course. The best way to cope with this is to do copious amounts of toe-touches all the way through the game. If it is too uncomfortable to get over into a bend, then squat on your haunches. This passively and very gently bends the spine around. It stretches out your lower back and disimpacts the vertebrae.

Loosening exercises followed by strengthening exercises before and after a round of golf will help to keep you playing. This means twisting the trunk as thoroughly to the right as you would swing the club to the left or vice versa. Also put in some sessions of full and energetic back-arching to counter all that concentration and crouching over a putt. The best thing to do is throw yourself into extension and release those pent-up joints.

RUBGY AND SOCCER

Rugby is bad for the spine. Together with parachute jumping, Rugby is the worst activity you can subject the spine to. Everything about Rugby worries me for the skeleton's sake. Although in truth it is probably the neck that suffers more than the back, but oh! how those joints get knocked around.

Imagine the impact on the joints of the skeleton of having one gigantic forward ploughing headlong into the midriff of another, both running towards each other as fast as their legs will carry them. Some of us feel it incumbent upon our joints to suffer traumatic injustice in silence forever. When we are in motor cars we try to avoid head-on collisions; the panel-beating is too expensive.

The other factor which contributes to Rugby damage is the heaviness and muscular bulk of the average Rugby-player. He is so solid that when he lumbers over the grass he almost dents the ground.

It is quite the opposite of the gazelle-like soccer-player. Picture the way the soccer-players leap through the air; no tackling, simply scoring points through light-footed co-ordination rather than by flattening some other poor chap.

Although it is true that the larger man comes off better from a Rugby tackle simply because his extra bulk rebuffs the assailant by bouncing him off, he suffers on the other hand because he is too heavy for himself. His over-powerful muscles keep his joints too bunched up and tight, not allowing them their full freedom. Trouble.

8

OTHER FACTORS WHICH

INFLUENCE A BACK PROBLEM

It is impossible to say what specific incidents trigger a back problem. We are all prone to trouble whether we are secretaries or stevedores, musicians or removal men. Backache happens to everyone.

But the common thread through all cases is that all of us have predisposed our spines to trouble by living a sloppy sedentary life interspersed with sudden bursts of over-energetic activity. The actual backache is the culmination of a developmental chain of events.

The back is a powerful but delicately poised mechanism, vulnerable to abuse. Some factors which may hasten the appearance of a latent back problem are discussed below.

AM I DEPRESSED BECAUSE OF MY BACKACHE OR IS MY DEPRESSION CAUSING MY BACKACHE?

Backpain is not easy to get rid of.

We all have only one back. If it is painful, there is no way of resting while you use another one. If your leg hurts, you hop; if your arm hurts, you put it in a sling and use the other one. Not so with the spine. It is on duty all the time, even during sleep when it will turn you over or otherwise re-arrange your sleeping position, time after time throughout the night. For every single second during a lifetime the spine is at work.

For this reason, back problems can be long-term and relatively difficult to treat. There are probably more man-hours lost to the industrialised Western world through backpain than through strikes. Treatment does not bring about instant cures. The longer the problem has been there, the longer it takes to get rid of it. Living tissue can only rejuvenate at a certain rate. Good treatment, combined with adequate rest periods between treatments and the abolition of all aggravating factors, will still take a few weeks.

During the entire time we are in pain we are disabled. At times it is not possible to think about anything else. It may be very difficult to keep going, let alone 'achieve' or 'excel'. The very backbone of our ability is broken, and that is depressing.

Pain is exhausting and with no relief in sight the prospect of the future looks grim. Apart from the here-and-now anguish of pain, the possibility that it could go on forever is a disturbing one. The anxiety takes many forms; depression is the most common.

If you are chronically depressed, it is very hard to fish you back out of the mire. No treatment will work if you are beyond emotional reach; if you are so depressed, you cannot even be roused to some expectation of recovery. You may have become locked in with your depression and your pain, one keeping the other going.

In practice one sees many emotionally wrecked patients who are close to being destroyed by their pain. At the time of the first consultation, one has the feeling that he can hardly rouse himself to go through it all again. He is weary of the expectation of relief. His replies to questions will be glib and unemotional. He feels convinced that he cannot give you any new leads by making the effort to search his mind for greater accuracy. Why should you succeed where everyone else has failed?

The demeanour of the person who is permanently in pain can appear strange. He may experience swinging variations of mood. At one time he may show frustration and despair when he may even appear insolent and hostile at the prospect of help. At another time he may appear withdrawn and restrained as if he dare not let it all out, lest he open the floodgates and dissolve into a collapsed sobbing heap before you.

Usually, breaking you free of the pain by treatment will restore you to your former old self. The depression lifts as the pain fades and uncharacteristic emotional behaviour vanishes. You had simply been brought down by the pain and now that it's gone you are feeling fine, free as a bird — optimistic and energetic.

Sometimes, however, you and your therapist just cannot

get rid of that pain. It will be worrying for the physiotherapist, who knows, by and large, from the way a back feels and behaves, how much pain it is responsible for.

Of course, we do listen to the patient's testimony about the pain, variable as that may be from one person to another. Perhaps you will continue to claim that you have pain. You continue to display the features of depression yet the therapist cannot find a valid physical reason to account for it. One side of the picture is there, the emotional one, without the other, the physical one. In these cases it must be rather unwillingly recognised that a patient's unrelenting anxiety is perpetuating the expectation of pain and the pain stays on. Sometimes it is even said that the pain is entirely a figment of the imagination. I doubt that there are many cases where this is so. Furthermore, if this were to be the case, one cannot say that the patient is not feeling pain. Pain is very subjective, impossible to measure objectively. One must believe a patient to be in pain if he, in his own mind, feels himself to be. Who is to say how much or little pain is imagined? And, if it is imagined, will it be any the less painful? It might be crippling.

Some patients grossly exaggerate their pain. It would seem that they suffer a confusing degree of pain compared to the relatively minor signs and symptoms that could account for the pain. Backache is difficult to quantify. No passer-by can tell if you are in pain, and sometimes we specialists are at a bit of a loss to know, too. However, there is a small group of people in the community who actually derive benefit from having a back problem. This behaviour may be prompted by the prospect of financial gain if there is litigation pending. It also may be prompted by a subconscious attempt on the part of the patient to gain attention or affection. He may feel that except for his widely publicised backpain he would be a faceless nonentity in the community. Alternatively, the patient may feel that the only way to rouse the partner or spouse out of his/her habitually indifferent attitude is to make him/her feel a sense of guilt or pity.

Such patients are extremely difficult to treat because they have no real incentive to give up their pain. They derive perverse pleasure through being unfixable; 'the nut that could not be cracked', or 'the back that dumbfounded medical science'. The problem has become part of them and their lives have adapted to accommodate it. In these cases the families need the help, not the patient. I am convinced that the number of patients in this category is small indeed in comparison to the genuine cases, but it is these people who give the general mass of back sufferers a bad name.

DOES TENSION MAKE MY BACK WORSE?

Tension plays a very big role in spinal pain.

If there is a joint problem created by a recent injury, the pain comes from pressure within the soft tissues created by the trapped fluid. Such tissues have the characteristic puffy swollen appearance.

If the problem is an older one, pain will come from perpetual stretching of the thickened or fibrotic tissues during normal functional activity. Either way, both types of joint problem will mean that the joint is tight to movement. The two bones making up the joint no longer hang together in a loose shuffling harmony.

Tension has the capacity to make matters worse because it tightens these already tight joints. This happens because tension increases the resting level of contraction in muscles. Instead of the muscles being limp and relaxed when they are not in use, they remain 'tense'. This creates a further joint-jamming effect which superimposes itself on the pre-existing tightness. The tension persists in keeping the two healthy joint surfaces pushed smack up against one another. Eventually the blood supply, and hence the nutrition through the joint, is slowed from a gush to a trickle. This causes the joint to become stiffer and more painful.

Even fleeting bouts of tension jam up the joints of the skeleton and increase symptoms coming from problem joints. The husband who is accused of upsetting his wife and making her backpain worse has something to answer for.

Long-term stress is even more serious. This alone can succeed in making a problem joint out of a trouble-free one, simply by keeping it smothered by layers of permanently unrelenting, tightly contracted muscles.

The leading problem is that the musculature loses the ability to relax. There is never complete recuperation of the muscles after activity spurts. There are no balming idle phases following hard work.

The mental spin-off of long-term stress is equally debilitating. Our judgement becomes impaired, our reactions inappropriate. We cease to be able to see goals and work towards them. Instead we toil away in a muddle where there is no beginning, no middle and no end to the day.

In this state, tension starts to gnaw away at the health. Sleep becomes fitful and we suffer through being denied the cleansing benefit of a night's rest. Increasingly, we lose the resilience to throw off more physical and emotional strains. Reserves are not replenished and we run down.

This is how disease creeps in; when the body's defences have been weakened by long-term stress. The joints are the first to suffer but they are not the last.

SHOULD I LOSE WEIGHT?

Popular opinion maintains that you should lose weight if you want to lose your backache. I don't think weight matters much at all. The skeleton can bear constant heavy weight without much complaint, especially the vertebral bodies. Bone itself, although it may feel very hard to you, is indeed only very hard soft tissue. It is pliable and bends a lot during activity. The vertebrae in particular 'sink and spring' with each heavy movement we make.

In fact, weight due to gravity, in combination with muscle activity, keeps normal bone healthy. Absence of gravitational pull on the bones as experienced by astronauts during protracted periods of weightlessness in space in one respect has proved the most enduring problem for the space scientists to crack. It appears that the decalcification of the bone that occurs in space is difficult to reverse. They cannot get the calcium back into the bones.

The everyday significance of this phenomenon means that normal stresses on bone, which include natural heaviness of the body plus all sorts of running, jumping and standing-still activity, keep the bones adaptable and robust.

Conversely, absence of body movement or a gross reduction of body weight results in demineralisation of the bones. This makes them brittle and inelastic. And the importance here is that, if bone springs less, the joints jar more. A happy medium between heaviness and activity is the ideal, and the joints will be slower to wear out.

While on the subject of calcium and bones and movement of bones making them stronger, the rate of healing of fractures is not an unrelated subject. We have found that gently moving the two opposing bone fragments at a fracture site will increase the rate of deposition of calcium within the soft plastic callus, the precursor of real bone. This means that the rate of repair of the fracture is faster and it is especially significant in cases of delayed union of a broken bone. It would seem that the age-old tenet of total, immediate and lengthy splintage of a broken bone in plaster of Paris may be about to go out the window.

Back to weight again. If you are overweight it is probably the other factors which go with being heavy which cause the harm. If you are fat, you are probably unfit. The big muscle groups will be out of balance, some short, some long and most weak. The important groups, most particularly the tummy muscles, will have reduced strength and reduced endurance. The skeleton will not be held trim and erect. You cannot effortlessly and subconsciously hold your belly in. Your thighs will be weak so that you have to haul yourself out of deep chairs or up a flight of stairs.

In brief, you will move badly in a sloppy fashion which is jarring for the joints. There will be 'postural strain' as you stand because everything starts to sag. As a consequence of inefficient movement, you will tire more easily. You have such a job to heave yourself about that you will tend to sit about more than a slimmer person does — heavy burdensome sitting in lazy postures, bad for the joints! The excess body load by weighing the skeleton down tends to accentuate bad postures. The poor posture strains the joints, not the pure weight load.

There are many fat but fit people. Look at those gargantuan Japanese sumo wrestlers. They will have no greater propensity to backache than you or I, because these other factors of unfitness or pure laziness do not exist. It is therefore quite possible to go on being happily overweight if that is what you want, as long as the general body performance is raised to carry that load. You may be able to minimise your backache losing weight. It undoubtedly helps the situation but does not rectify the cause. To do that, you need to clear up the mechanical problem responsible for the pain and then tone up the muscle support system to hold the spine in correct alignment. Thereafter you can stay as fat as you like, if you don't die of a heart attack.

If you are overweight but manage to get a bit fitter, the improvement in strength and in heart/lung function will make it easier to get around doing everyday things. The weight will start to drop off just because you are moving about and doing more. Unwittingly you will make yourself slimmer without even trying. This accounts for the common observation amongst dieters that in the early stages of the diet nothing seems to be happening. Then suddenly, after this latent period, weight loss gathers momentum without any appreciable change in the dieting format.

Dieting, that subtlest form of torture, need not be so drastic if you concurrently do more activity to burn the weight off. So many hapless dieters starve themselves on half a lettuce leaf and a cardboard biscuit. They have so little energy to work on that they drag themselves about all day flopping from chair to chair quietly getting fatter and fatter through the lack of activity! A most unfortunate stalemate and a very common state of affairs.

Dieters need to recognise one important fact: reduced intake of food lowers the metabolic rate. This is an in-built precautionary measure to stave off disaster but it means that the less we eat, the less oxygen we consume and the less able we are to be active. Our activity palls because our 'fire within' fades and this leads to an increase in fat reserves. Beware of stringent dieting!

WHAT SHOES SHOULD I WEAR?

There are two important things to remember about shoes: the height of the heel, and what the heel is made of.

The higher the heel, the more it tips the body forward in front of the line of gravity. The pelvis is thrust forward, the low back over-arches to bring the weight of the upper body back behind the line of gravity again, so in effect all the spinal curves become exaggerated. Pain is never far away. There was a fashion for so-called 'Earth shoes' designed with the heel lower than the forefoot. These employ the opposite principle to encourage better posture and a healthier spine. They are quite a good idea.

However, just as important as the heel height are the shock-absorption qualities of the heel, for minimising the impact on the spine when the heel strikes the ground. The softer and more rubbery the heel, the better. Crepe rubber is the best; wood is the worst; and wood with metal caps under the heel is fiendish.

City gents do not like crepe rubber soles too much. They do not go well with the pin-striped look. 'Sorbothane' sole-inserts are a good alternative. However, they do not go as well in women's shoes, especially the higher ones, since the insert tends to creep down to the front of the shoe and runkle under the toes. An insert may also make the foot rest too high out of the shoe.

I will insist on any patient undergoing treatment for a particularly nasty back problem wearing shoes with crepe rubber heels. I would also like him to wear them thereafter if he will.

SHOULD I WEAR A SURGICAL CORSET?

Except in rare circumstances, which I will describe in a moment, these contraptions are positively the worst thing you can do to your back.

If there is one message I have tried to get across in this book, it is that movement is therapeutic. Although it might hurt to move, there are good hurts and bad hurts. Most are good, and move we must. Movement begets movement. The more we move a joint, even a painful one, the better it moves. Pain is usually the result of poor mobility from malfunctioning joints.

Corsets came into vogue because we — doctors, physios and everyone else offering treatment — could not think of anything better to do. The poor patient was having such a dreadful time getting about with that back, better strap him into a corset to help the poor spine stay upright. Never mind what was wrong; just hope that it goes quiet in the meantime.

To encase the low back in a corset is a stupidly short-sighted solution. It simply makes the spine stiffer; brittle and vulnerable, ready to be jarred by more and more trivial bumps and bangs. Spinal tolerance to shock is steadily reduced.

The short-term gains of a corset are:

• A tightly worn corset can 'unload' an intervertebral disc by reducing the intra-discal pressure to the same degree that it is unloaded when we are lying down. In the instance of bulging-disc problems, corsets, as a short-term measure, come into their own.

• In cases of severe inflammation of one of the spinal

joints, there is an initial reduction of pain because the joint is kept quiet.

• A sagging belly is pulled in closer to the line of gravity thereby reducing the forward drag on the low back. This reduces back-pain associated with too deep a hollow of the low back.

• In the event of severe spasm of the back muscles, it is useful to support the spine with a corset to allow the over-active muscles to relax.

The long-term disadvantages of a corset are:

• Increasing propensity to injury as the spine becomes more rigid;

• Increasingly weaker tummy muscles as the artificial support allows them to go into complete retirement.

The patient who arrives for treatment for the first time wearing his friendly corset is usually a tricky one to manage.

For months, even years, he has been faithfully following medical advice never to leave his bed without it. It usually looks dreadful, belts and buckles everywhere, usually very grubby because it is never off. He feels naked, vulnerable and frightened without it. He feels his spine will do something dreadful without that corset, and the sad truth is that it probably will since it has ignored its own natural resources of strength and suppleness for so long.

You must be weaned from your corset before you can start getting better.

The way to get you better is to mobilise the stiffness out of the spine and then gently to exercise the tummy muscles to restore them to full strength so that they can support the spine.

In the circumstances where corsets do have a short-lived role to play, their advantageous effects are derived from the tightness of the garment rather than from its rigidity.

You may have noticed that professional weightlifters wear a very tight belt around the waist. The purpose of this is to pull in the waist and greatly increase the pressure inside the belly. This 'unloads' the spine and reduces the risk of straining the back during a heavy lift.

To be useful, surgical corsets must employ the same principle. The waist-belt must be hitched in very tight and the steel stays inserted down the back of the corset should be thrown away.

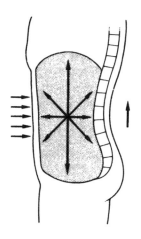

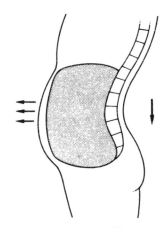

55 The bracing effect of a corset increases the intra-abdominal pressure which 'lifts' the spine off the discs.

WOULD A TIGHT BELT HELP?

Employing the same principle, there are some spines which can be greatly helped at a certain stage in their recovery if you simply wear a belt, the wider and tighter the better. This is for the back which has been very laid up and is just getting going. A belt helps most when you are up and about walking, especially if you are walking on hard concrete or stone surfaces.

The back may harbour a collection of problems: degenerated discs at multiple levels, facet joint arthropathy, weakness of the spinal musculature, spasm of the spinal musculature, inelasticity of the neural matter — the works! Backs such as these are abnormally sensitive to impaction shock of the foot-fall on hard pavements. They feel weak and stiff and also exhibit a marked reluctance to bend.

But their cure lies largely in regaining the ability to bend! The discs suck in fluids by bending which recoups their health and vigour. And the muscles are strengthened by bending which shores up the internal strength of the spine. However with a fragile back all this takes time and this is where the belt comes in. Because with a nervous patient tentatively gaining ground, it can be nothing short of disaster to hurt the back at this stage. You may need short-term abdominal bracing to get you over the hump. A corset is too much but wearing a tight belt for a while might just fill the bill. The increased intra-abdominal bracing buffers the spine and frees it to go about its business.

IS BENDING BAD FOR ME?

No. Bending over in a deep full sweep and up again is unquestionably the greatest treat you can give your spine. Bending keeps the spine young.

The old directive of 'back straight, knees bend', faithfully carried out by hordes of patients young and old, is the single most misguided, erroneous principle ever to be propagated. This simply perpetuates a stiff brittle spine, and that you do not want! Besides, there will always come a time when you have no option but to bend — usually an emergency — like catching a falling plate or some other completely reflex action. If your spine is not well accustomed to bending confidently, a trivial everyday incident can cause havoc by demanding something of that brittle spine that should be second nature.

Of course, if you are to bend and lift a heavy weight such as a suitcase or a bag of shopping, then it is better to lift like a weightlifter with the back straight and bending the knees (see 'How Should I Lift?' later this chapter). But for the average bend — say, to get the detergent from under the sink, to put socks on, to pick up a handkerchief from the floor — you absolutely must use your spine.

That bend gives the discs a drink. The nucleus, inside the intervertebral disc, is composed of a colloidal jelly which attracts fluid. The nucleus thereby entices fluids in to nourish itself. But this process is greatly helped along by full expansive movement of the spine. By sitting down, standing up, stretching, twisting, bending, etc., a squash-release-suck effect is created to drag fluid and food into the disc from the rich bed of blood in the centre of the vertebral bodies above and below the disc.

It is important to say that a variety of different directions of bending is desirable because this minimises the risk of weakening one particular part of the back wall of the intervertebral disc which would allow a bulge to be forced out with greater ease. But, on the whole, bending as a pastime suffers undeservedly from a bad reputation.

It has been shown that patients confined to bed in hospital for non-back-related reasons lose disc-height on X-rays taken before and after their confinement. Because their discs were deprived of the benefit of generous movement and therefore their ability to feed themselves, they in effect shrank from malnutrition.

Full and generous bending, because it is the grandest movement the spine does, also keeps the ligaments and all the soft tissues supple and stretchable; it keeps the facet joints at the back of each vertebra well oiled; it keeps the spinal cord free and slippery in the spinal canal and it keeps the spinal nerves elastic like strands of cooked spaghetti, free to pull out of the spine as the tension tightens on the sciatic nerve with each bend forward.

Bending is a little more tricky if you are right in the middle of a bad flare-up of an old problem, especially if you know there is a degenerated disc in evidence. However, although it is still imperative that you should bend, the initial twenty degrees tilting forward from vertical should be undertaken with care. The stomach muscles should be braced (maybe with a belt), sucked in like a greyhound, even with a hand gently restraining the tummy, as you pass through the 'weighted-bending' phase. This is the critical stage of the movement where a problem disc will tend to pinch a bulge out the back of the disc wall.

Once the movement passes this phase the lumbar spine goes into the 'hanging' phase, the particularly valuable part, when the real benefit of the bend begins. The back of the segment is opened out, which disimpacts the facet joints and, just as valuably, creates a suction effect on the sagging back wall of the disc which drags the bulge inwards.

If you do not feel secure enough to bend, fearing that the back will go into a sudden muscle spasm, then lower yourself down into the full bend by climbing down your thighs taking a lot of weight through your arms (see diagram 44.1, Chapter 6). When you are down there, then hang. It does not matter whether the knees are straight or slightly bent as long as you really stretch the spine. As you hang there make small oscillating bounces. The way to return to vertical is to suck the tummy in, tighten the buttocks to rotate the pelvis under, and wind up to vertical from the base of the spine upwards. If the back feels weak and vulnerable and threatens to go into spasm as soon as this new bending venture is attempted, then prepare the spine by bending it in the completely unweighted position, lying on your back on the floor and bringing the knees to the chest.

Another means of making the exercise less alarming is by strengthening of the 'intrinsic' back muscles (see diagrams 53.1, 53.2, 53.3, Chapter 6). This will provide the spine with much needed, almost instant strength so that it loses that unnerving feeling that it is about to give way.

Bending over and staying bent as in gardening is another story. This is a strain. It is an impossible leverage for the muscles to cope with for any length of time, so they get tired and start to ache with the fatigue. This also stretches the soft structures of the spine too much over too long a period of time. The more you return to the upright position, the less strain there will be. To garden you should be squatting or kneeling, making sure to keep the tummy braced so that the spine does not sag forward.

HOW SHOULD I LIFT?

Lifting in the workplace has done a lot to focus the collective mind on the problems of backs, not least because of the cost to industry. Over the last decade in particular, there has been a lot of debate: What is a safe weight to lift? Should we bend to lift or keep the back straight? Should we lift with a hollowed back or with a rounded one? In short, what can we tell our workers so as to keep them in work and out of the courts?

It's really quite amazing how a back can lift, bearing in mind that this involves bending over to the floor and then correcting to vertical while at the same time carrying a load. Like a half-shut knife, opening out to straight. Sensational.

The action is best understood by watching the techniques of professional weight-lifters, because they demonstrate in a pure form, what heavy lifting is all about.

The key factor in successful heavy lifting is powerful intra-abdominal pressure. As a weight-lifter bends over and contemplates the weight, he signals the start of the lift by a deep, stout inhalation. This fills the lungs with air and causes the diaphragm to descend into the abdominal cavity. By the abdominal cavity reducing volume, it increases pressure. This shores up the spine within and thrusts it upright.

This pocket of pressure under the diaphragm is exactly like a hydraulic sack which buoys the spine aloft and un-bends us from a curled position to upright. It is rather like a child's tubular paper whistle which will un-bend and straighten as it is blown full of air. Professional weight-lifters know well the value of heightened intra-abdominal pressure as seen by their use of 'kidney belts' to enhance their performance.

The importance of intra-abdominal tone in a non-lifting state is well illustrated by the unfortunate decline of polio-myelitis victims who have suffered paralysis of their trunk muscles. Because their musculature lacks tone, the torso in time will gradually crumple around itself. The muscles are unable to contract and build up enough abdominal pressure to push the spine aloft and the spine topples over. The result is an increasingly marked spinal deformity.

Back to the art of lifting. When we are bent over to take the weight from the floor, the spine is relatively safe. It is locked by virtue of being at full stretch. All is well to take the first heave. The trickiest part comes when the weight is airborne and the lifter is halfway up. Trouble sets in when the spine itself comes off full stretch, when the vertebral segments can shift and shuffle under the burden of the heavy weight.

At this point, the successful lifter unconsciously ensures that the spine does not develop a disastrous wobble by almost imperceptibly rolling the pelvis backwards so that the

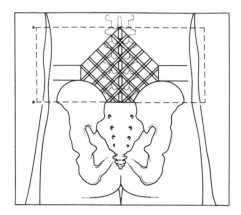

1. When the muscles
   are inactive, the lattice
   is deeper and the
   spine separates.

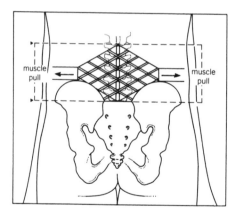

muscle pull

muscle pull

2. As the muscles pull out
   to the side, the
   lattice flattens and the
   spine 'clamps down'.

*56 The action of transversus
abdominus and internal oblique
muscles on the latticed thoraco-
lumbar fascia.*

lower back becomes taut and humped. In the process the stomach forcibly contracts.

But this is often the stage where the lift fails. Technically speaking, the load comes off the ligaments and is transferred to the back muscles. It is the critical transition where the spine flicks through from a full stoop to the full arch and the point when the back can 'rick'. It can be prevented by powerful balloon pressure from the abdomen below. With the spine now off the stretch, intra-abdominal pressure elongates it from within and stops it wobbling. This momentary phase in effect 'rolls' the torso over a sprung spine, enabling the strongly contracting back muscles to safely take over.

Incidentally, an important recent advance has paved the way in unlocking one of the chief mysteries of the lifting back and I need to go on to explain this: Researchers were confused when their mathematical calculations appeared to disprove the ability of a fine, streamlined human back to lift. Judging by the known muscle-contributers, the power to straighten under load did not seem to be there. That was until they found another two muscle groups to help! The tranversus abdominus and the internal oblique, were observed to actually help straighten the spine and thus perform the opposite action to that which they were previously thought to do. This means that some of the missing straightening power, over and above that provided by the long back muscles, was now recognised as coming from the unlikely source of the stomach or side-trunk muscles.

It seems their contribution is twofold. Firstly, they tighten transversely around the girth, thus pressurising the intra-abdominal cavity, which we know to be valuable. But more importantly, by their attachment to a lattice-like sheet of tissue (the thoraco-lumbar fascia), which in turn attaches to the backward projections of the spinal vertebrae, they assist directly in straightening the spine. As we will see in the section on 'Pushing' below, by tugging laterally at the edges of this broad sheet of tissue, these two muscles cause the lattice to shrink in height as it is stretched out sideways. This has the effect of approximating or bringing together the individual vertebrae of the spine in just the same way as when we straighten. Far from tipping the spine forward and causing its small knobs to move apart as it elongates, the action of the muscles and the fascia draws the backs of the vertebrae together.

The very same action of the human lattice regulates the free fall of the torso as it tips forward in bending. This is again why it is so important when bending always to pull the stomach in as tight as possible; it tenses the thoraco-lumbar lattice which retards the rate at which the vertebrae move forward off one another.

This underlines once more the importance of tight stomach muscles for lifting, bending or even sneezing for that matter! It also explains why serious weight-lifters pay just as much attention to stomach strength in their work-out regimes, as they do their backs and legs. They recognise that without a stomach as hard as steel they will hardly be able to lift a fly! Well almost.

To revert to lifting in the workplace: with repeated heavy lifting it is the intervertebral discs which suffer the brunt of the destructive forces. As we have seen in the section on disc degeneration and prolapsing (see diagrams 13 and 14, Chapter 3), discs tend to suffer wear and tear at their left and right back corners. If we picture a disc as a clock face, the greatest area of wear and tear corresponds to 4:30–5:00 and 7:30–8:00. This is because these 'corners' are the parts of the rim which are most pinched in rotatory movements. This is important because virtually every movement we make involves rotation. Movements of the human body are never pure. Even passing the salt involves a certain degree of twist. It gives us animals our own peculiarly 'living' way of doing things, as distinct from the mechanical up-down movements of a robot, for instance. It allows us to address objects face-on rather than at a less manageable angle. This is particularly relevant to lifting. We have to bend to the side as we go down and come up, to get out of the way of our knees.

When we go to bend forward, there is a 'pay out' of the muscles on either side of the spine which act like large elastic cables, gradually letting go and allowing the spine to tip forward. Once we have grasped the weight to be lifted, these same cables contract and help pull the spine back up straight. This exerts compression on the spine, particularly on the nuclei of the discs which tend to squirt backwards and affront the back wall of the discs. The back wall is even further subjected to shock if the nucleus is partially dried and the rim is forced to bear a greater than normal load. If we add together the compression and the torsional strains of lifting, you can see that the forces of destruction on a back and particularly the discs, are great.

That is why lifting in the workplace needs to be carefully controlled. As far as injuries are concerned, not much difference has been found between a stooped lift with a round back or a lift with a straight back. The critical factor is the strength of the stomach. Another, or course, is the closeness of the weight to the body. The further out in front of the body the weight is carried, the harder the job.

Lifting movements should be as varied as possible, bending down to the left a few times and then to the right. Try to intersperse the lifting routine — again as much as the working environment can accommodate — with some form of 'pause activity' such as spinal extension (see diagram 40.5, Chapter 6). If the nature of the job means that repetitive lifting can only be carried out in the one direction, the pause activity should concentrate pure rotation movement in exactly the opposite direction to that of the lift. This is important, as it will maintain mobility of both sides of the skeleton, thereby reducing the likelihood of overuse and strain on one side. Pure side-flexion pause activity is often as beneficial as the rotation and spinal extension — that is, standing with your legs planted well apart and bending over sideways, running your fingertips down the outside of the thigh to the knee and below. This movement should also accentuate the opposite bend to that employed in the lifting action. You should also try, if the work situation permits, to avoid lifting directly from the floor. The height of the surface from which the object is taken is important. Generally speaking, the higher off the floor the better, the optimum height being around forearm or elbow level. Any higher will mean that it is harder to get at and that the weight has to drop into the arms, posing the risk of jarring the back. If the object is heavy, you can brace your hip against the structure on which it rests and take it cleanly in your arms without putting any undue strain on your back. The height of the surface where you will put the object down is equally important. Keep your stomach braced at all times and your eyes on where you're putting the load before you actually lower it. If the lifting you have to do is heavy, repetitive and long-term, wear a kidney belt — or quit!

If you carry medium weights, such as babies, my considered view is that more backs can lift than think they can lift. In fact, within reason, too many people with a problem back do not make it do enough. A back will never be normal if you do not insist it does normal everyday things. A bit of lifting is very beneficial, especially if it is done in an unhurried and controlled way with the tummy braced. It strengthens the spine and helps break that stalemate of stiffness/weakness which is the commonest cause of ongoing trouble.

It may be useful to get into a stride or lunge position when lifting a medium weight. This means that you in effect swoop down on to the weight and scoop it up, making the lift a full and dynamic movement rather than a harried stab of movement from above. A deep lunging movement also means that the big joints like the hips and knees, which are designed for load, are involved in the movement instead of just one willowy spine working like a derrick. Keep the tummy braced.

It is quite possible that the back may be a bit sore and stiff after some easy lifting, but that is not a bad thing. Don't be thrown by this and rush straight back to bed. The average back sufferer is too easily frightened by the worry of another 'attack'. This anxiety and the consequent tension hasten the arrival of another attack, which might never have happened. If the back is a bit sore after lifting, do some gentle rolling, some toe-touches and then some sit-ups (see diagram 37, Chapter 6). Then some more lifting tomorrow.

Lifting an awkward weight, like lifting a heavy weight, also has its risks. For that reason there are a few fundamentals that must be followed. First, get right up close to the weight with back absolutely straight, knees bent. Get a very secure finger hold of the weight. Make sure the helper is going to lift at exactly the same time as you (lots of back injuries occur when the other fellow drops his end). Lift by straightening the knees. Tummy braced.

Featherweights and light weights should be collected up from the floor with one full sweep of the spine down to the floor and up again (see 'Is Bending Bad for Me?' this chapter).

I know this flies in the face of just about everything you ever heard about back care, but you just try it! Stiff upright rigidity is dangerous.

WHAT IS WRONG WITH PUSHING?

Pushing is a problem. In my experience there is no other activity more able to bring down a normal back. And it can be something so simple like pushing a shopping trolley or mowing the lawn! One particular muscle which works rigorously during the act of pushing is the transversus abdominus. The fibres of this muscle wrap transversely around the sides of the lower trunk between the bottom of the ribs and the top of the two hip bones. The action of the transversus is such that as it contracts, it tightens around the waist like an elastic cummerbund. However, at the back of the torso the muscle attaches itself to a broad flat expanse of soft tissue consisting of diagonally placed fibres resembling a lattice. As its outer end is pulled taut by the contracting muscle, the lattice expands laterally but shortens longitudinally. Since the other end of the lattice attaches to the lumbar vertebra it means that whenever the transversus abdominus contracts the lumbar vertebrae are telescoped together. This is a superb piece of muscular enterprise. It means that whenever such a contraction takes place during the act of bending or pushing, the spine 'clamps itself down' and resists forwards and backwards shear. The lattice steadies or tempers these otherwise risky movements by its compressing action. Sure enough, if you push hard against an object you will feel the side of your waist harden with the effort. The only hitch is that excessive effort in pushing may create too much telescoping and bring to light an underlying lumbar problem. Pushing is often the last straw.

Unfortunately, the shape of the facet locking mechanism also works against the interests of the spine during pushing because it encourages spinal compression. These bony catches act in such a way that they lock against each other when we bend forward and this prevents each vertebra slipping off the one below. As we bend forward and until the lock engages, the upper vertebra slides up and forward on the lower vertebra. But when we do the opposite movement — such as occurs in pushing — the upper vertebra slides back and down the one below bringing the two vertebrae closer together. Thus backward shear tends to jam the spine down upon itself.

And whatever is wrong with the spine, it will be aggravated by this sort of compression. For one, the discs are squashed and if any are degenerated they will be sorely aggravated. And as for the facet joints, they will be annoyed too by the excessive overriding caused by the compression.

The reverse movement of backward shear — that of one vertebra being pushed forward on the one below — may account for the uniformly pleasing results of central mobilising pressures as a treatment technique (gliding the vertebra forward from behind), whatever other movements the spinal segment lacks.

This manoeuvre in effect slides one vertebra forward on the one below, thus disimpacting the two bones as the upper one runs up the slope of the bony catch below. These central pressures, as we physios call them, are the single most effective therapeutic measure to employ on a painful back.

The results from a few quick pushes and pokes to a problem vertebra are astonishingly good. Would the good Lord

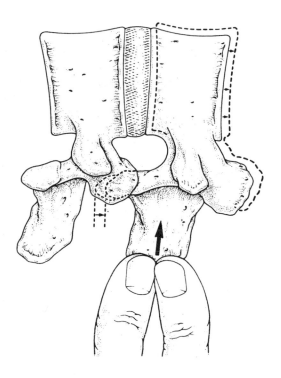

57 The simple 'sliding-up' effect of pushing on a lumbar vertebra. Two adjacent vertebra are disimpacted.

have made it any other way? Cavemen didn't have access to injections and image intensifiers and CAT scanners and the rest of the shining armoury of chromium gadgetry. If a chap had a spot of backache, he probably got his mate to give his back a bit of a rub or maybe even got him to put his heel into the painful spot, and that was that. Modern science has made us all too fragile with ourselves, too much in awe of what might be wrong and what must be done to put us right.

HOW SHOULD I CARRY THINGS?

If you are faced with one large weight, make it into two smaller equal weights, carried in both hands, tummy braced. Do not let the weight pull you down so that the tummy protrudes and the shoulders droop. Have frequent stops.

If the weight is a smaller, more manageable size, then it is best carried clutched to the chest. Never carry a weight out from the front of the body as if to stop it soiling your clothes. The leverage created on the spine will immediately create strain on the low back.

Perhaps we should take a leaf out of the book of the people of the Indian subcontinent. All the women carry on their heads, which totally eradicates any leverage strain caused by carrying, and the men carry large weights with poles over the shoulders so that the full brunt of the weight is carried by the ribcage. We are crazy to use our arms.

HOW CAN I COPE WITH LONG-DISTANCE TRAVEL?

Except for trains with sleeping compartments, we have yet to evolve a means of travelling long distances any other way than sitting up. This is all very well if you want to read or write or look at the view but it takes a heavy toll on the spine. Sitting makes the spine compress longitudinally so that it bunches up like a piano accordian, rarely getting a chance to elongate and suck in a fresh breath of air.

When you think about it, sitting is a very odd thing to do. Folding up in the middle like that and perching the tail on a convenient surface. Spinally speaking, squatting is a better alternative due to its poised rather than flopped nature. With squatting we are kept aloft by co-contraction of the paired trunk and leg muscles which is not the case with sitting. With a back of the seat for support, we flop. The abdominal wall lets down as the girth slackens and the belly spills forward over the brim of the pelvis. The hydraulic sack qualities of the abdomen let go and the rib cage sags. This weighty collapse compresses not only the abdominal contents but it compresses the spine. The spine vertically settles down upon itself and squashes the discs. One of the earliest pieces of bio-mechanical research showed that the pressure within the discs is increased during sitting. And, that as long as we remain sitting and the pressure stays on, fluid is forced out of the discs. Relatively speaking, our discs dry out. Like a dense sponge in a vice, water oozes out. This loss of discoid fluid under vertical compression is known as 'axial creep'.

As more fluid squeezes out of the disc, like air out of a car tyre, the nucleus deflates and the spine settles down on the fibrous disc rim. The spine becomes brittle and cramped and is compromised in rebuffing impact from below, compression from above and jolts from the side. This is all very well for a healthy spine but not so good if it isn't. If a spine is riddled with stiff links like the random scatter of rusty links in a bicycle chain, it is easy to see how long-term sitting can tickle up an existing problem or bring a dormant one to the fore. Over time, sitting squeezes drier spots drier. This is not only the discs but all the soft, water-filled tissues holding the spinal segment together.

Most rehydration occurs spontaneously at night while we are asleep, as long as we are lying down. The discs stealthily imbibe fluid and we actually grow a centimetre or so, as we lie there. During the day we usually depend on body movement to interrupt the shrinkage. The everyday activities of bending, reaching, stretching, twisting, standing up, sitting down, all exert a 'squash-release-suck' effect on the discs which pulls in water and boosts the spine's stature.

Sitting travelling for long periods, say in an airline seat, brings the two factors together, the loss of fluid from the discs because of the raised intra-discal pressure and the inability to recoup the fluid because of the forced inactivity. Long-distance lorry drivers probably have the worst of it, with an incidence of back trouble four times the national average and probably triggered by heavy lifting between long spells at the wheel.

A third phenomenon comes into play during extended periods of sitting and this relates to the general 'squidgy' nature of the tissues in and around the spine. The soft tissues of the spine are extremely vascular, that is they have an abundant blood supply. The tissues themselves, ranging from the bone, disc, cartilage through to ligament and muscle, all have a high water content. You might say they are water-logged, even bursting with fluid. And this explains incidentally, why inflammation and its simultaneous swelling always cause such havoc, particularly in the back.

These fluids can be pushed into pooling pockets at the back of the spine if it stays kinked or bent over in one position for too long. In the case of a traveller sitting slumped for hours in a seat, or a carpenter crouched hammering nails all day, the front parts of the spinal joints are 'milked' as the fluids squeeze through to the back. They escape from the compression to collect on the other side where things aren't so tight but then they can't get back. They become trapped as a bloated wedge of fluid. This accounts for the difficulty we all experience in getting upright again after long periods bent over — sitting or gardening or vacuuming or tinkering over a car engine. The collection of fluids on one side of the spine acts as a block to the spine realigning itself up straight. This is known as 'creep in flexion'.

An acute back flare-up will often present like this too. The sufferer stands bent forward and miserable. Any attempt to get straight will cause a sear of pain and the legs to crumble. Usually it is muscle spasm which has locked the spine crooked so that pooling occurs but the pain will not ease until the spine has been gently brought straight and the tissue fluids have balanced their distribution. The way to do this is described in Chapter 6 (see diagrams 40.1 to 40.5).

But a more common back condition is the older drier back. It grumbles from time to time but really plays up when it has to travel. Its discs are dry and have lost bounce. They are harder to squash flat and then harder to puff up again. All the other tissues are drier as well, less elastic, less able to absorb shock.

Or, you might be a fit young buck with one level in your back behaving like this. Just a single joint which has been previously damaged; a rusty link in a glistening chain. This is the commonest condition I see in clinical practice — an otherwise mobile and elastic spine hampered by one stiff link in its midst. Even one segment misbehaving in this manner can cause the sort of 'old man's back' syndrome so often the source of such dismay.

It's obvious from all this that any back with a problem is going to be severely taxed by long-distance travel. A rusty spine, or a solitary rusty joint in a healthy spine, whatever. The sitting is going to sorely deprive it of its lubricating juices. You see it so often in an aircraft when people pull themselves out of their seats and stand for awhile, trying to coax their bent frames upright.

However, the good news as far as travelling is concerned is that although you cannot possibly avoid 'axial creep' — the slow settling of the spine down upon itself — you can avoid 'creep in flexion' by at least attempting to sit properly. If you avoid slumping in a heavy and hopeless C-shaped curve, you will minimise its happening as far as possible. It may be worth remembering that keeping your seat-belt on helps to prevent your bottom sliding forwards and your shoulders from slumping.

Another adverse effect of travel comes from prolonged vibration. Vibration speeds up the flow of fluid out of the discs. Air travellers may fare better than those in a train or car simply because the vibration is less but there are other problems with planes, not least the reduced cabin pressure. Though the plane may be flying at an altitude of 9,000 metres, cabin pressure is maintained at a level of 2000 metres. This is considerably less that the air-pressure at sea level and is one of the reasons why our feet swell.

So what with the inertia, the vibration, and the settling and hooping a travelling spine suffers, it clearly needs some help. There are a few things you can do.

Some of them you do instinctively anyway, like arching in the seat and stretching the arms in a subconscious attempt to disimpact and reflate the spine. But sometimes you'll see passengers disregard these signals and straight away haul themselves out of their seats, only to find that their backs won't straighten. Then they compound the damage by reaching up to get baggage out of the overhead lockers.

I have treated many a back which has come to grief at this point. A spine which is not only compressed but set lopsided in a semi-rigid hoop is hardly in a condition to extend itself upwards in one jerk, not to mention saddle itself with a barrage of baggage coming down from the lockers. And the last straw that breaks the passenger's back, so to speak, comes at the baggage claim. The big bags create real mischief. Usually they are so heavy they can only be carried one at a time and the killer is yanking them off the moving track.

You can minimise the ructions by following a few simple precautions. Needless to say, they all revolve around *movement*. Basically, the more you move the better — though not at the expense of your fellow passengers' peace of mind. Don't wriggle around in your seat or clutter the aisles by touching your toes. There are other things you can do sitting unobtrusively in your seat that are every bit as effective.

The most important thing is your long-term sitting position. Try to keep your lumbar spine in 'mid-position', neither too scooped in a hollow nor too slumped in a broad 'C'. Of these two extremes, the latter is the more tempting to adopt. Avoid this by keeping your bottom as close to the back of the seat as possible. The further it slides forward, the further it takes the lower back away from supportive contact and the more you flop. Stuff a small airline pillow into the transitional area of your spine (see section on 'Chairs', Chapter 9) and this will stop your spine from creeping vertically down the back of the seat. Apart from neck support, this is the most effective use of these pillows. However, most people put them too low and end up almost sitting on them. Keep monitoring your position and if you find yourself creeping forward shift backwards again. 'Walk' backwards on your buttocks to get to the back of the seat or lever yourself back by using the arm-rests. Either action will dramatically alter the pressures on your spine and break it loose from its impaction.

Slowing of the circulation, in particular the venous return of blood up from the legs to the heart, is another consequence of lengthy air travel. Partly the result of reduced cabin pressure which facilitates the pooling of blood in the lower legs and partly the result of forced inactivity, the business of getting the blood around the system and back up to the heart is an up-hill job. The kinking of the large veins of the pelvis as they traverse the front of the hip joints is another impediment. The angled hips obstruct the flow of blood and create back-pressure in the venous system. Sitting with the legs crossed adds to this. A fourth impediment to easy circulation is the sitting pressure on the buttocks and the backs of the legs. Simply sitting on them, blocks the passage of blood through the tissues. This is the chief nursing hazard in caring for the incapacitated and the elderly. Deprived of a healthy flow of blood, flushed through with every beat of the heart, the tissues quickly break down. 'Bedsores' develop from the pressure of body weight. Though travellers are not prone to such extreme dangers, the process is the same. Blood flow is hampered when passing through pressure areas.

To help all your joints, your circulation, your digestion and your peace of mind while travelling, you need movement.

Probably the most effective means of restoring juice to the discs and bounce to the lower vertebrae is to rock your spine back and forth as you sit in the seat. You can do this in two ways. The first is by humping and hollowing the lumbar spine in and out of a concave and convex curve. The more exaggerated the movement the better: you have been stuck too long. Imagine as you rock over the discs that you are activating them like a vertical row of bellows, sucking fluid in and out. Emphasise the concave phase to counter all those hours spent slumped. Do this by thrusting your fists into the small of your back and reinforce the forward movement by pushing with your hands. Push forward three times for every hump backwards.

The other way to open and close the discs is by the sideways movement, though the available freedom in this direction is much less. Rock from one buttock to the other, at the same time bending your trunk sideways as you lift your weight off the seat. This exercise requires quite a deal of tummy strength and incidentally is very effective in shrinking the waistline.

These two exercises help to 'prime' the discs in readiness for more adventurous tasks like wrestling with the baggage. But another standby is a sitting version of the exercise shown in Chapter 6, diagram 43.1. This involves lying down more on the seat. Although this puts you in something of a slump, it partly takes the weight off the spine. In this semi-recumbent position, bring one thigh up onto your chest by holding your knee with both hands and bounce it. (Impossible to do in a skirt!) Do one knee and then the other and repeat the procedure many times; you cannot overdo it. You can also exercise the calves and lower legs. Sit squarely in the seat with your legs bent at an obtuse angle and feet planted firmly on the floor. Lift both heels and point your toes. Then reverse the action. Press both heels into the floor and pull your toes back as far as they will go. Repeat over and over again for as long as you can endure before cramp creeps into the muscles of the shin.

This reduces the swelling in the feet by the alternate pumping action of the muscles at the front and back of the lower legs. When a muscle contracts, its fibres shorten and its bulk thickens, pressing against the stocking-like casing of the skin of the lower leg. This pumps the interstitial fluids back into the circulation towards the heart. This muscle-pump action operates all the time, assisting the heart in shunting the circulation around the body. Easy to see why gentle activity helps the workings of the heart.

Finally, when you stand up, do it carefully. You have been impacting a long time. Use your thigh muscles to push you up and brace your stomach. If you have only partially unkinked your spine with the humping and hollowing exercise, you will need to do a bit more straightening once you are upright. Push your hands into the back and prise yourself straight. Then arch backwards a few times, especially before you start carrying.

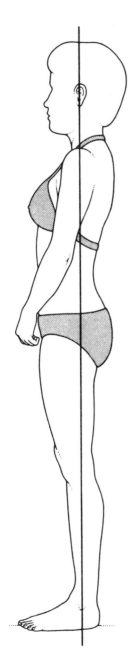

58 Ideal posture.

9

YOUR OTHER QUESTIONS

ANSWERED

With an estimated nine out of ten — or even more — of the population at some stage likely to suffer from backache, you can be sure that however miserable your back has made you, you are not alone.

From my experience in handling all kinds of backs and the people to whom they belong, I have been able to identify the questions back sufferers are most anxious to have explained. I have presented them to you as they are presented to me.

WHAT IS GOOD POSTURE?

Good posture is the best way for the skeleton to hold itself upright to carry its weight most effortlessly. This means in practice that, in side-view, you have the centre of gravity passing in one straight line through the ear, the middle tip of the shoulder, the middle of the fourth lumbar vertebra, the middle of the knee and just behind the outside anklebone of the foot.

If there are pronounced abnormalities of posture, the movement mechanics of spine, the limbs and the head become more laboured. The weight of the body is not managed so well; stresses caused by movement are not tolerated so easily.

Faulty posture over a long period of time will chronically strain the skeleton and ultimately cause pain.

The four most common types of bad posture are:

1. Increased lumbar lordosis, 'the hollow low back';

2. The thoracic kyphosis, a rounded thorax and shoulders which may also be associated with a rounded low back

as well, or may be associated with a lumbar lordosis;

3. The 'too straight back' where there is not sufficient thoracic curve;

4. The 'poke neck' where the head is carried too far in front of the body, causing that nasty aching pain in the base of the neck and across the shoulders.

Changing a bad posture is not easy. It is, after all, the habit of a lifetime. Posture is also intimately related to psychological factors and therefore unlikely to be corrected by physical measures alone. However, if bad posture can be improved, it makes the world of difference to one's sense of well-being.

The best possible treatment approach if it is recognised that faulty posture is the cause of pain is, first, manual mobilisation of the various stiff spinal segments so that the spine is then freed to assume a better stance. Thereafter you should carry out some of my stretching exercises to loosen all the tight muscles, tendons and ligaments which had adaptively shortened and in effect 'held' the bad posture in place. Finally, you need exercises to strengthen those weak muscles which, once they are more powerful, will be able to hold the spine in a better alignment.

Here are some stretching and strengthening exercises to help counteract the four main faulty posture types.

(1) The Hollow Low Back

Stretching/loosening: Knees to chest in the lying position and touching toes in standing position, to stretch out the tight muscles of the low back.

Lying on the back, pulling each knee up alternately to bounce it hard on the chest while leaving the other leg down on the bed, stretches tight hip flexors which through being tight keep the front of the pelvis permanently tipped forward (see diagram 45, Chapter 6).

Strengthening exercises: To strengthen the loose muscles of a tummy which is stretched, weak and not providing an adequate retaining-wall support for the spine, do thirty sit-ups daily.

Gluteal exercises by their increased strength help pull the tipped-forward pelvis around to a more normal inclination: either pelvic raising in the lying position with the knees crooked and bridging the pelvis or doing squats in the standing position.

59 *Pelvic bridging increases the strength of the muscles of the buttocks. Their added strength helps to reduce lumbar hollowing.*

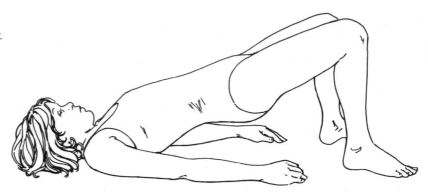

(2) The Round Back

Stretching exercises: The most important stretching exercise is to lie on the floor with a pile of pillows under the ribcage so that as you relax the lumbar spine sinks deeper down into a gently arched curve totally unlike its habitual forward slump.

This can be progressed by doing the same thing also in the prone position and pushing up on your extended arms to arch the spine backwards (see diagram 40.4, Chapter 6). It can also be done while standing.

The next exercise is chiefly aimed at stretching out the thorax, which by being tight and hunched over is adding to the general picture of a hoop-shaped spine.

Lie flat on the back on the floor, lift both arms and attempt to place them on the floor above the head. Keep the elbows straight and close to the ears.

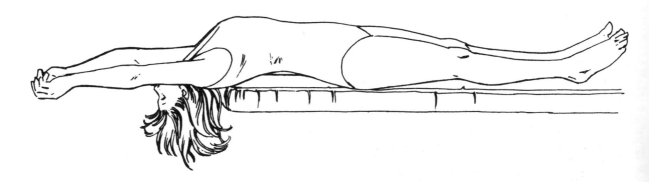

60 *The thorax stretch to 'undo' habitual working postures.*

This exercise can be made more effective by doing the same thing off the edge of the bed, the edge of the mattress under the apex of the curve of the thorax. In that position bounce the arms back in a gentle oscillatory fashion to stretch the spine gently. Strengthening exercises: Lie face down on the floor over two pillows stacked under the belly. Hands behind head, lift head and both legs back off the floor together. This strengthens the 'long back extensors' and helps to hold the spine more upright (see diagram 48, Chapter 6).

(3) The Too Straight Back

Both the above sets of exercises will help here, but the emphasis should be on loosening rather than on strengthening.

(4) The Poke Neck

The best type of exercise for this type of abnormality is the generalised spinal stretch which comes about when you lie flat on the floor on your back and swing your legs up over your head and rest the toes on the floor behind your head. In yoga this is called the 'Plough' and it is a wonderful experience for the entire spine. The exercise can be progressed by lowering the knees down astride the head to rest beside the ears.

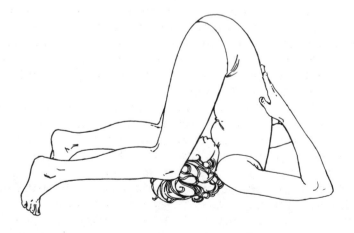

61 By stretching the spine, especially between the shoulder blades, the 'Plough' helps rectify a poke neck.

This exercise is always difficult and must be done very gently to start with. It may be months before you can get the knees on the floor beside the ears. Take it slowly!

WHY IS LYING DOWN SO UNCOMFORTABLE?

If lying down is painful, it is probably what you are lying on! A soft bed is usually the culprit (see 'What Is the Best Bed?' next section).

By and large, lying down is the most comfortable position for a painful back. The spine is in repose, relieved of all postural stress, so it can relax and that will reduce pain. The intra-discal pressure is at its lowest lying down, greatest sitting, and somewhere in between when standing. The spine actually elongates in sleep. This comes about for two reasons: first, the natural curves of the spine which have increased slightly through the day, weighed down by tiredness and hard work, flatten out with rest; secondly, relieved of the pressures of weight-bearing, the discs actually suck in fluid in small quantities. This expands the disc and raises you in height.

During the day, there is a net flow of fluid out of the disc. The fluid is actually squashed out and the spine imperceptibly 'settles' down on itself — especially after a lot of casual sitting or standing about. We then feel that irresistible desire to stretch and bend the body to 'puff up' the spine again to make it feel more comfortable.

All this being so, back problems rarely worsen while you are lying down. However, there are exceptions.

In severe cases of facet joint arthritis (sometimes called arthrosis but more usually osteo-arthritis), that common or garden variety of arthritis which we all have in differing degrees after the age of sixteen, there will be discomfort after lying for too long. You will feel the urge to get up and move about. Doing just that will relieve you of your pain for a while. You will feel relief after changing position but find that you are only comfortable in the next static position for a while. Then you must get up again or just change position. Getting up and moving about stirs the joints out of their sluggish torpor and eases any discomfort.

Whatever the cause, if you feel progressively worse after lying down it may be that the muscles in spasm have gone into even greater spasm. Muscles automatically go into a protective cramp as a reflex to save a sore joint underneath being further pulled about. Problems develop when the stiffness created by the muscle in spasm makes the joint more sore by not allowing it the benefit of movement.

The best thing to do to break this vicious cycle is deliberately to stretch the muscles in order to release their hold. Do this as soon as you wake up before attempting to pull yourself out of bed with your rigid low back.

Lie on your back and gently bring one knee up towards the chest. Pull it up on to the chest and release. Repeat that many times, a hundred times if necessary, just gently bouncing. Then do the same with the other leg.

It is not really manageable to try to lift both legs together. They will be too heavy and it will be less easy to keep a relaxing rhythmic bounce going.

After that has loosened you off a bit, get down on to the floor for spinal rolling (see Chapter 6).

Remember that lying face down in bed will give almost any back a pain. It is true that this is a favoured position for a lumbar disc problem, but this is a very rare cause of low lumbar back pain.

All backs, except those kept habitually in a rounded slump, are strained by sleeping face down. This is because the lumbar spine lies slung between two supports, one the ribcage and the other the pelvis. With muscle relaxation induced by sleep, the lumbar spine quietly sags into a deep hollow. This is fine if all the joints are healthy and elastic, but a joint which is not free to 'give' will get hurt all over again. The weight of the spine tends to tug at this unstretchable link. As a consequence you wake with a nasty sore back, cast in a hollow shape. It is very difficult to get up, so you roll over and lever yourself up sideways, usually accompanied by an assortment of grunts and groans. There is no hope of getting your socks on.

WHAT IS THE BEST BED?

I always find this a difficult question to answer, because it all depends on two variables: your weight (and your partner's weight) and the degree of stiffness of your spine. There is always debate over whether the best bed is the one that allows your spine to go into a hollowed arch or, the opposite, a slumped curve, because of what those two extremes of posture will do to a problem disc. Since problem discs are such a relatively rare source of pain in the back, it seems a fruitless argument to me.

Bear in mind, too, that we change our sleep position literally hundreds of times a night, so that any one position is of no particular importance because we so quickly move out of it. In short, do not worry what a bed does or does not do to all the various different pathologies that might affect a back.

The important thing about a bed is that it keeps the spine from lapsing into extremes of any posture. In sleep the spine needs to be firmly supported. The support must maintain as nearly as possible the healthy curves of the spine. A soft sagging mattress will bring on pain in a problem back because, whether sleeping on the back, front or side, it will allow the spine to sag. The stiff joints, unfortunately, cannot 'give' and sag as well, so they will be strained in the process. You will wake up stiff because the muscles have gone into protective spasm. You will be stuck, stranded like a beetle on its back, having to roll over and lever yourself up sideways to get out of bed.

However, just to confuse the issue, in some cases sleeping on a very firm mattress is not too comfortable, either! All too often the poor patient, fed up with having back pain and heeding the advice of a thousand do-gooders, goes out and spends a small fortune on the latest orthopaedic masterpiece, only to find that when he gets it home it is impossible to sleep on. As a general rule, the stiffer the spine, the less able it is to adapt to a very hard bed. If you are extremely stiff at every spinal level, then you will probably be more comfortable in the interim, before your spine has been made sufficiently supple again, to sleep on a medium-hard mattress. At least then there is some contour support rather than the two unresilient obstacles, the spine and the mattress, fighting it out till dawn.

As a general rule, the bed for you is the bed that does not collapse in a big hole when you sit on the edge of it. It should comfortably take your weight, and be firmly springy. The more healthy and elastic the spine, the more support it needs in sleep and therefore the harder the mattress needs to be.

IN WHICH POSITION SHOULD I SLEEP?

Sleep in any position that is comfortable.

Most backs, but particularly those which sit habitually with an increased lumbar hollow, are made more uncomfortable if you lie face down in bed because the hollowing is increased. On the other hand, if you have a rounded low back which sits slumped, you need to lie face down and be passively forced out of that permanent stoop.

If you are in the middle of a nasty back flare-up, then probably the most comfortable position is on your side and cuddling a pillow, 'a Dutch wife', and another pillow between your knees with the knees drawn up.

Another comfortable position for sleeping in, though not necessarily in bed, is particularly useful if you have just 'done something' to your back (see 'Have I Put My Back Out?' Chapter 3). Lie on the floor, bend the legs up. Rest the calves on the bed or sofa. The hips should be at ninety degrees. If the support surface for the calves is too low, then build up under the calves with cushions so that the support is very slightly lifting the bottom off the floor. The effect of this is twofold. First, by slightly lifting the weight of the low back from the floor the spine gives itself very gentle self-traction which separates the jarred joint. Secondly, rounding and therefore stretching the low back in this way inhibits muscle spasm from becoming too intense.

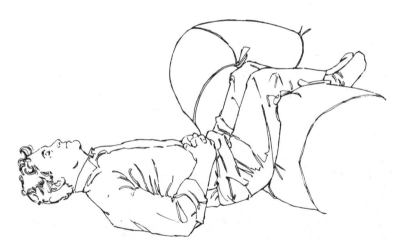

62 An excellent position for relieving an acutely painful back.

Before getting up from this position, gently tilt, swivel and roll the pelvis. This presses the jammed segment into the floor as the movement rolls over it and helps loosen it.

WHY IS SITTING SO UNCOMFORTABLE?

Sitting, although providing rest and recuperation for aching feet and legs, is not a good time for the back. The intra-discal

177

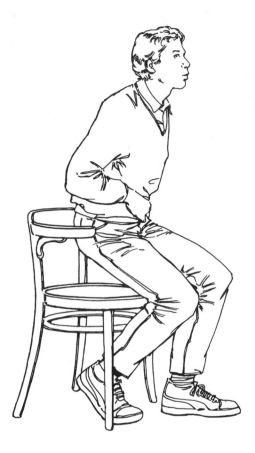

63 *The best way to rise from a seat is to brace the abdomen with a firm restraining hand and use the thighs to elevate the body.*

pressure when you are sitting is much greater than when standing. The spine is much more jammed up when the base of the spine is resting on a seat. If there is an unhealthy bulging of the intervertebral disc wall, it will be apt to increase. Therefore, sitting will be painful.

The variation on this theme is the back which is just fine while your are sitting but gives an excruciating jab of pain as soon as you go to stand up.

There are two theories about what goes wrong here.

The first is that the pain may well be produced by a ballooning disc. Pressures within a disc are at their greatest when the vertical spine is tipped forward by twenty degrees, at about the point where the sufferer feels that nasty jab of pain.

Pain on rising from sitting, however, can also indicate an instability in the integrity of the spine caused by a weak link. When the spine tips forward as it does to initiate the movement in getting up from sitting, a shearing strain is imposed across the lumbar spine. A weak joint will be stressed by this strain.

Pain in both cases can be minimised by bracing the tummy muscles before rising. In the case of the problem disc, this reduces the forward inclination of the spine so that it stops short of the twenty-degree point and thus avoids pain. Here, one rises more by elevation using the powerful thigh muscles than by simply lurching forward to get the centre of gravity over the feet.

In the case of the unstable segment, the act of bracing the tummy before getting up from sitting raises the intra-abdominal pressure so that it works like a hydraulic sack. It exerts back pressure on the spine to prevent its vertebrae slipping forward.

The other state of affairs which makes sitting uncomfortable is complicated.

Sometimes, as a result of very nasty inflammation of one of the joints of the spine, all the soft-tissue structures nearby, everything except the bone itself, are affected by this inflammation.

All the soft tissues involved in the inflammatory processes ooze clear lymph fluid. This may also include the loose membranous sack which wraps around the valuable spinal cord itself, the dura. The fluid tends to get gluey and sticky as it lies about; not pumped away in the course of normal activity because you are in too much pain to move! Eventually the stagnant fluid becomes stringy 'adhesions' which tether the delicate dural membrane to the inside wall of the bony spinal canal.

After the acute backpain has passed and you are up and about, not feeling much pain from the joint, this dural tethering is barely noticeable. Gentle activities that do not stretch the spine will not provoke any pain from the harnessed dura.

However, with prolonged sitting, the spine tends progressively to slump deeper and deeper as you get more tired and heavy. As the back bows into the slumped position, the spine increases in length and the cord inside the canal stretches rather like a pulled-out concertina. This has the effect of drawing the cord in from the side-walls of the vertebral canal, thus drawing the spinal nerves back in through their exit-canals as well.

However, in the presence of dural tethering, many little hair-like adhesions are binding the dura to the wall of the spinal canal rather like the hairs of Gulliver's head were pegged to the ground by the Lilliputians! The dura gets tugged and thereby irritated when it is not free to move normally as the spine bows. The common signs of dural tethering are back and/or leg pain after lengthy periods of sitting, typically after long car journeys or aeroplane flights.

The only way to treat this problem is to use the same treatment principles applied in treating all other problems of inelasticity of soft tissues — that is, gently and persuasively stretching it to regain its normal stretchability.

The way to do this is to bend the body in two at waist level either by standing, trying to bring the head to the knees (see diagram 44.2, Chapter 6), or standing swinging the leg of the affected side forward in repeated straight-leg high kicks.

With the head-to-knee exercise the forward movement of the head and spine tends to pull the spinal cord 'upwards' inside the spinal column thus freeing it. The leg-kicks pull the spinal nerve tight in the leg, thus pulling the spinal cord 'downwards' in the spinal canal, which frees it in that direction.

When both exercises have become relatively pain-free both should be tried in combination. Standing on the good leg with the 'bad' leg supported on a low stool, knee straight, the head is gently forced on to the knee of the supported leg and bounced up and down until the tight pain eases.

As this becomes less painful, the supporting surface for the 'bad' leg is raised higher and higher from the floor (or, more simply, start the exercise with the 'bad' leg supported on a low chair and progress to supporting it on a high kitchen

64 Straight-leg kicking is the most effective means of freeing a tethered nerve root.

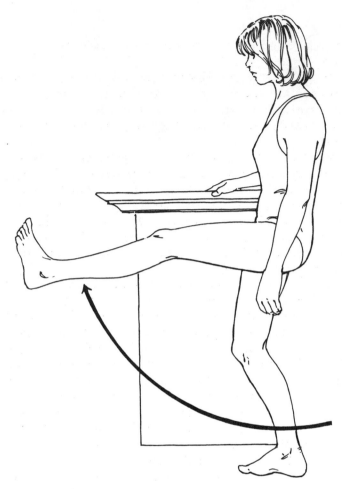

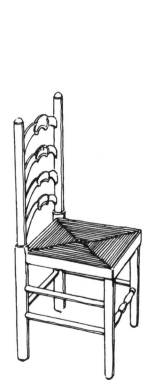

65 The worst chair – a straight back at right angles to a straight seat.

table). The process is gradual and must not be hurried. Nervous tissue and its protective covering are very intolerant to stampeding tactics.

WHAT IS THE BEST CHAIR?

The same idea about what constitutes a good bed applies to what constitutes a good chair.

You want a chair that effortlessly maintains the healthy curves of the back. When you sit, your spine is stacked upright upon itself supporting its weight against gravity. A little support in the right place can make all the difference between a comfortable chair and an awful one.

Sitting becomes uncomfortable when the chair allows the lumbar spine to fall into extremes of posture, either too hollowed out or too slumped. Both facet joint and disc problems, the two most common causes of pain from the back, will be aggravated by chairs which accentuate the curves of the spine.

In the case of facet trouble, caused usually by degenerative change — arthritis — the joints complain fiercely when they are put in their close-packed position, all bunched up. However, they will complain just as readily when they are on the stretch. They are bunched up when there is too much extension or hollowing of the lumbar area, but they are stretched open if the spine is too bent over on itself, slumped forward in a hoop. Degenerated joints adapt badly to both extremes.

The problem disc also does not sit comfortably when the spine is subjected to extremes of lumbar postures. If the spine sits stooped, the back wall of a problem disc will distend. This adds insult to injury if there are symptoms coming from that disc. However, a problem disc will appreciate any chair which forces a hollow into the low back because this will take pressure off the back wall of the disc.

Here is a run-down of what makes a good and a bad chair. The worst chair is one with a completely straight back at right angles to a completely straight seat. Sitting on one of these for any length of time can be purgatory! The rounded, more protuberant part of the spine, the thoracic kyphosis, is unable to arch back naturally over the lumbar spine, because the chair-back is in the way. The whole spine above the lumbar area is pushed forward in front of the line of gravity and it fails to sit easily upon itself. Stress falls at the 'transition' area of the spine, that point between where it arches inwards in the lumbar area and where it arches outwards in the thoracic area. Here the muscles have to work overtime to keep the body from slumping forward. After a while they begin to fatigue and start to ache.

If the spine is not able to carry itself in a balanced equilibrium, with just as much weight sitting behind the line of gravity as in front, then it will ache, even if the back is usually healthy. How awful to sit in a chair that makes even a healthy back ache! And there are plenty of them about, usually in restaurants. The only way to get comfortable on one of these fiendish chairs is perch one's self right on the front edge of the seat and recline so that only the transitional curve of the spine rests against the chair. However, it is a very crumpled way of sitting and impossible to continue for any length of time.

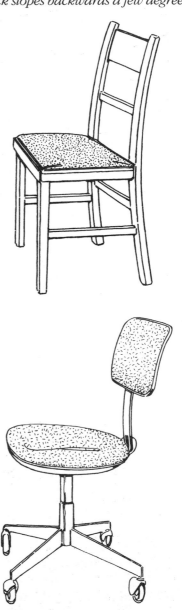

66 A more comfortable chair – the back slopes backwards a few degrees.

67 The typist's chair with the upholstered pad which nudges into the low thoracic spine, the transitional curve, as it descends in a sweep towards the hollow of the lumbar spine.

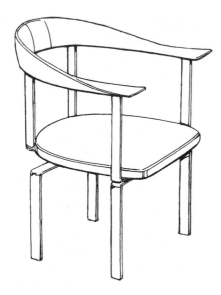

68 *The dining chair with its back support encircling the body at lower-rib level.*

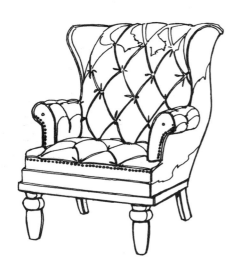

69 *The bulky, uncontoured chair.*

A chair-back which slopes backwards a few degrees beyond the vertical so that it lies in line with the transitional curve as it sweeps up from the lumbar region is so much more comfortable.

A particularly bad type of chair often has a straw base scooped out in the centre so that the front frame of the chair neatly cuts into the back of the thighs in the most uncomfortable manner. The only way to relieve pressure is either to cross the legs, which is bad for the spinal alignment (and terrible for varicose veins), or to hook the heels over the chair-rungs at the front of the chair, which does terrible things for the posture.

The best type of functional all-purpose chair is the transitional bar-support chair. These are commonly seen as typists' chairs. They are ideal where the occupant does not need to lean forward a lot to work. The back-support section of these chairs consists of a soft but firm upholstered pad which nudges transversely across the spine quite high up, just about under the back of the lower ribs. If the transverse pad is connected to a hinge, the arrangement is even more satisfactory. It not only allows the occupant the freedom to arch backwards to stretch after heavy periods of concentration, but its variable angulation backwards allows the spine to sit on the soft pad and thus off-load some of its weight.

The back support, contoured to the transitional curve, even tends to lift the spine as it passes back over the centre of gravity. As a consequence of the partial unloading of the heavy weight of the torso above, the lumbar spine (which so readily tends to lapse into lazy heavy postures, either completely slumped into a 'C' curve or the other way, into a hollow back with the tummy resting on the knees) will tend to hang below the support bar in a much better alignment.

There is a satisfactory variation of the typist's chair manufactured as a dining-chair. This has a back support which encircles the body at lower-rib level continuing around the sides of the chair as arm supports.

If the chair is well padded it helps, as does a slight bevelling of the back section which sits in contact with the spine.

Unfortunately, most chairs of the transitional-bar design fail to extend up high enough and therefore rarely do any real supporting.

Excellent as a typist's chair is, it's a bit skimpy. You would not find any top executive-type sitting in one behind his huge executive desk. He wants a chair as expansive as his desk. The bulky, uncontoured chair, a heavy chair of the highly stuffed variety, is commonly seen as this sort of desk chair. They are old-fashioned in style, well padded, with a gently sloping back away from a well-sprung seat and bulky arms which are at exactly the right height to allow the occupant to rest his elbows to take weight if he wants to. Chair-arms are much better upholstered if you are going to spend a lot of time in the chair, because if they are comfortable they can bear up to 22% of body weight.

The common fault with bulky chairs is that in their overall grand design they tend to have a seat which is too deep. The average individual feels inclined to pad out the seat behind his back with pillows to provide some support.

The latest in chair design are the contoured chairs but they are not all necessarily suited to the human spine. There are good and bad contoured chairs; both are expensive. The good type is the one in which the seat is very slightly tilted downwards from front to back, and the back-support consists of a firm, protuberant upholstered pad making good contact with the spine primarily at the transitional curve of the spine. It is good because the pad 'lifts', as discussed earlier, and the slightly back-tilted seat tends passively to correct any hollowing of the lumbar spine by pressing the occupant in closer contact with the support pad at the back.

There is no real need to support the spine beyond the transitional curve. However, if you do want a high chair for some reason, then another firm pad nudging gently underneath the back of the head and massaging the base of the skull is a good idea.

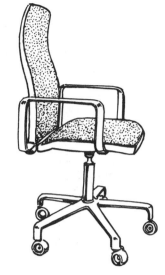

70 The well-contoured chair has a softly contoured protuberance which extends well up the spine of the seated occupant. Most contoured chairs are rendered useless by the pad being too small and too low.

71 The average economy-class aircraft seat provides no support for a sitting spine.

72 The soft-foam sofa; impossible to sit in and impossible to get out of.

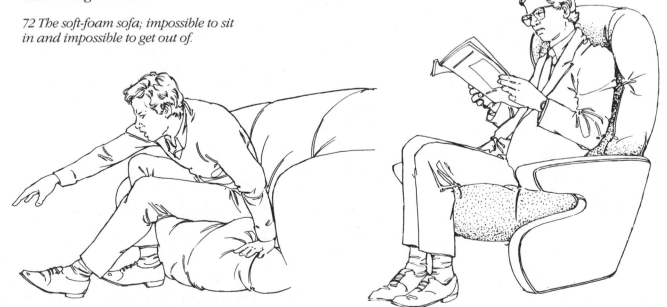

An ordinary bulky chair like the one described earlier is infinitely preferable to one which has been poorly contoured. Badly contoured chairs too readily conform to the non-tired shape of the sitting spine. They do not provide enough support because they do not sufficiently over-accentuate good spinal alignment. They fail to lift and support the heavy chest and head. They often have a too deep thoracic curve so that unless you are a huge man with a great barrel chest you get swallowed up in the hollow, especially if the protruding neck-pad is too high, which it usually is. The old economy-class aircraft seats were often badly contoured. So are Concorde's; it's a good thing the trips are so short.

The soft, squashy and deep chair or sofa that lets the whole spine collapse in one continuous 'C' bend needs mentioning here because it is so bad. You are better not to sit if it means sitting on one of these! They are usually made entirely of foam with no proper base. They typically cause an ache in the low back, even in healthy individuals, because they encourage the spine to bear weight in such an unnatural way. They are particularly bad for a low back prone to disc trouble. By allowing the spine to adopt a curled position, the vertebrae above and below the disc pinch together at the front and gape open at the back. You get up from this 'easy' chair and you can hardly straighten. You are forced to get about for a minute or two fully bent forward. You must push your hands into the small of the back and force it inwards to get yourself upright again.

Here are a couple of general rules on good seating.

1. The seat part must not be too deep. If it is, it will be impossible to sit back comfortably with the back well supported and the feet resting squarely on the floor. In extreme cases, the front edge of the seat will press into the back of the calves, and the feet will barely reach the floor. The low back sags into a deep uncomfortable curve because there is no back support to push it upright.

2. There is an optimum height of the seat above the floor: the chair should put the knees just slightly lower than the hips. If the chair is any lower, so that the knees are higher than the hips, the low back will slump into a 'C' shape. It will also mean that the chair is too low and it will take too much effort to get up out of the chair.

If the seat is too high off the floor so that the knees are substantially lower than the hips, particularly if the feet

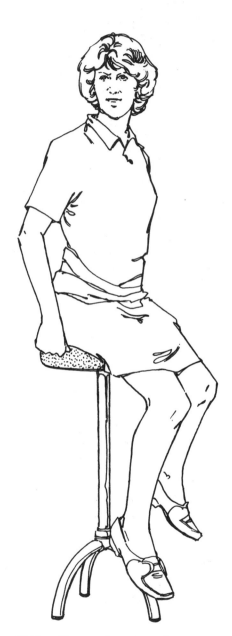

73 *The effect on the spine of two heavily hanging legs is to pull the lumbar spine forward in an uncomfortable arch.*

cannot even touch the floor, you will be very uncomfortable.

Discomfort is created by the dragging effect of the strong hip flexor muscles which connect the front of the lumbar spine to the top of the thighs. The front of the spine is pulled forward into a hollow by the tension in these large and powerful muscles.

Finally, one of my favourite chairs is the 'Balans' chair, made originally in Scandinavia. These are cleverly designed to tip the pelvis forward so that one takes weight through the knees on small upholstered pads. The occupant of the seat takes very little weight through the bottom. Thus there is little of the jamming-up effect induced on the spine in the sitting posture. The other, secondary advantage is that in this position the spine automatically assumes the almost perfect 'S'-shaped alignment of perfect posture, much the same as one assumes otherwise by squatting on the haunches. Just try squatting for a bit. You will quickly see how pleasingly the spine hangs in this position.

There are two disadvantages to this type of chair. First, they encourage the lumbar spine to hollow forward, and for backs which get pain by doing this, sitting will be painful. This effect can be partly minimised on the adjustable chairs by lowering the seat further towards the floor, thus lowering the bottom almost on to the heels. Of course, the heels do not actually take the weight of the bottom, but it becomes a strain on the knees, not to mention the ankles. This is the second disadvantage of the chairs.

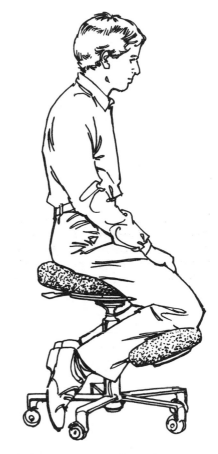

74 The ingenious Balans chair.

WHY IS STANDING SO UNCOMFORTABLE?

The commonest reason why standing is uncomfortable is that it tends to accentuate a bad posture and that will increase strain on a poorly functioning joint (see 'What Is Good Posture?' at the beginning of this chapter).

Casual sauntering about or leisurely idle standing which does not demand a great muscle effort allows the spine to sag deeper into its natural curves.

But, although you may have pain when standing, you might find that you are completely free of pain while bustling about with great purpose. More activity demands that the postural muscles all work harder. This keeps the spine held taut and well controlled, free of the temptation to sag and become painful.

There is another specific condition where backpain is much worse when standing. It is associated with an overwhelming desire to sit down to relieve that pain. It is called spondylolisthesis — the slipping forward of one vertebra and the spine above it which it is supporting, off the front edge of the vertebra below. It happens when the bony negative and positive 'hooks' at the back of each vertebra, the facet joints, are broken or otherwise made incompetent, thereby failing to hold the spine snugly intact.

75 Spondylolisthesis, where the natural bony hook at the back of the spine is rendered incompetent and fails to prevent a natural inclination of the uppermost vertebra to slip forward.

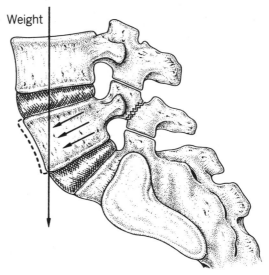

Weight

Spondylolisthesis commonly occurs at the two low lumbar joints L.5 slipping forward off the sacrum or L.4 the second-lowest vertebra slipping forward off L.5. The reason for the high incidence of slip at these lower two joints is that the lumbar lordosis, the hollow in the low back, is greatest here. Therefore the angle of the slope on which the vertebra sits (the sacral angle) is the greatest. The hollow is more pronounced in the standing posture, but is almost completely straightened out in sitting. Because the sacral angle is relatively large in the standing position, there is a pronounced shearing strain induced which brings about pain as it stretches all the soft-tissue structures trying to restrain the slip.

The treatment of serious spondylolisthesis is surgical spinal fusion of the slipping level, especially if there is severe pain and even more especially if the degree of slip is increasing.

If symptoms are not marked, spondylolistheses do well with manual mobilisation of the vertebral segments above the slip (which have usually become stiff as a secondary compensatory development of the instability of the joint below), followed by the intrinsic spinal stabilising exercises to bind the weak link together again as strongly as possible (see diagrams 53.1 to 53.3, Chapter 6). In some cases of quite marked slip — half a centimetre or so — there may be no symptoms at all. You may go through life with this and never know about it.

IS SEX BAD FOR MY BACK?

I have always had a feeling that the patient who asks me this question secretly hopes that I will throw up my hands in horror and forbid all forms of sexual activity under pain of death. This patient wants me to excuse him/her from the travails of the bedroom.

However, the truth of the matter is that a little gentle sex is about the best thing for a bad back, especially if you are on top. Yes, very definitely very superior therapy. But if the act is too aggressive, with lots of heavy banging around, then you will inevitably thump your own and your partner's spine around something awful.

It is, indeed, a clever trick of nature that the skeletal muscles used in the act of coitus are the same two very powerful and important groups which maintain the frame in an upright posture and also propel the frame along in the process of walking. I do not have to tell you that these two functions are the first two fundamental requirements of man: to stand upright and to get about. Believe it or not, sex comes third!

The first muscle group is the strong gluteal group — the buttocks — perhaps the strongest group in the body. They are in action all the time we are upright. A low-grade level of contraction keeps us from folding up at the hips. As well as this they have the added action of thrusting the body forward on the straight weight-bearing leg in the support phase of walking.

The second muscle group is the abdominal group, the tummy muscles which, fortunately for most of us, can succeed in life without being as strong as they might. Their primary role is to hold the belly in and act as a brace to prevent the spine from protruding forward at lower spinal level. Their lesser role is to rotate the pelvis and bring it

187

around from the hollow-backed position to the hump-backed position.

The best action for both partners during intercourse is gentle rhythmic rolling of the pelvis where the spine humps and hollows alternately. The pelvic action is supplied by the tummy muscles and the thrusting action is supplied by the gluteals.

Strictly speaking, anybody who has a slack tummy is sure to be a lousy lover. You'd better take a look at yours.

IS HOUSEWORK BAD FOR MY BACK?

The problem with housework is that it is exacting and tiring without being energetic enough. It means long periods of toiling at awkward angles, usually with the shoulders stooped and the head bowed, but the whole activity is not dynamic enough. The skeleton with its elastic joints is not treated to the benefit of grand-scale flourishing movement.

Modern gadgetry has made things easier but not easy enough. The good romping stuff has been taken out so that we are left with the paltry ungenerous activity, so commonplace of our lives today, which is tiring but which is not exuberant enough to keep us fit. In fact it even does the opposite.

In the pursuit of an explanation to account for the increasingly frequent complaints of non-specific aches and pains, perhaps vague in nature but possibly crippling, usually from younger members of the workforce and especially those involved in tedious and repetitive manual work, a modern syndrome has been evolved. Its name: repetitive strain injury (RSI).

If you think about it rationally, it is hardly surprising that in some instances the human skeleton makes known its objection to the use which machines increasingly put it to. It is yet another flaw in the machine-dominated world in which we live. The trouble is we have not yet realised that like those machines we, too, go wrong and like those machines we, too, need maintenance.

It is the price we pay for our dependence on machinery, and the machine-operators pay the price for the rest of the community.

Just imagine for a moment, if you will, the wear and tear subjected to the joints of those women who stand beside a production line and repeat the same movement day in day out, month after month, year after year. It is the lack of generosity in the movement which causes the trouble. The repetition is another thing. But if there were more flourish and flamboyant romp there would be more blood supply and lubrication reserves called into play to take care of the incessant physical demands continually in force upon the tissues.

As it is, the joints become locked in meagre patterns of severely limited movement, and the muscles and tendons start to chafe and fray like the fibres of old rope worked back and forth relentlessly over an old and rusty pulley. Of course, if you then add to this the complete picture of lethargic leisure hours, poor diet with too many cigarettes and cups of tea, you get your aches and pains sure enough.

As for housework, three types spring to mind as the most demanding on the human frame: vacuum cleaning, ironing, and making beds.

Vacuuming is a problem, especially if the machine is a tubular one that you pull along the floor behind you. It involves staying bent for long periods of time, pushing the nozzle across the floor, and we all know that sustained bending is bad and so is pushing (see 'What is Wrong With Pushing?' Chapter 8). To help matters a bit, reduce the suction as much as possible so that it is easier to push the head across the carpet. It helps, too, if you can push the head away from you with the face of the nozzle at an angle to the floor so that it is not effectively applying suction. Then flatten the nozzle down on to the floor to pull it back to you so that it sucks only as you are pulling it towards you. Make the rigid tubing as long as possible so that you can push from hip height. Try to keep as upright as possible as you work.

The old-fashioned upright cleaners are better for backs than the cylindrical type. The reason for this is that their action is different. They have a circular rotating brush which beats the carpet and gets all the dust airborne. Once it is airborne it is then sucked up. This, together with the fact that the head runs on big wheels, means that it is much easier to push, not glued to the floor by the suction. These machines are also easier to use because one stands more upright to push them, though they are not as good at getting into corners and under beds. The choice is yours.

Ironing is a problem, too, because it involves such laboured long hours standing there. Inevitably, the spine will sink down into deeper and deeper curves as the tired tummy muscles gradually give up the battle of keeping the spine in trim. My advice is either to sit on a high stool to iron or to get a small box about twenty-three centimetres high to put on the floor under the ironing-board so that you can put one foot up on it. The box should be quite robust so that you actually take weight on the upper foot. This position will take the sag out of the low back by rolling the pelvis back and pushing the spine into a hump rather than a hollow.

Making low beds is also a problem, especially double beds. It is not so much the bending down that causes trouble as lifting the mattress up and stuffing the sheets and blankets underneath. The action of leaning across the top of the bed to throw the bedding up near the pillows is also taxing if the reach is supported by a typically soft abdomen. In this position the poor back acts like a derrick. It is a classic way of straining the back.

The best way to make a bed is to crouch beside it on your haunches, not on your knees because there is better capacity to use the leverage of the strong thighs to make the activity more dynamic. Keep the tummy braced and do not hurry. This is also the position to use to clean the bath.

Whatever housework you are doing, it will be taxing. The best way to minimise the long and tiring sessions of strain is to punctuate them with energetic bursts of stretching movements, particularly into extension. Especially when you feel fatigued and achy, drop everything and fling yourself into a backward arch with the head back and both arms stretched out above the head. Do it several times. It works wonders.

WHY IS MY BACKACHE WORSE BEFORE MY MENSTRUAL PERIOD?

The alteration in hormonal balance before a monthly period results in pre-menstrual fluid retention. Women often complain of feeling uncomfortable and bloated. This is because they are not eliminating body fluids as readily as they would do at other times. The fluid collects in the soft tissues. The joints do not escape this effect, so that any joint which is swollen and painful anyway will become more so. The worst times are the few days immediately preceding the period, but in some women it can gradually increase from the middle of the cycle up until the day or so before the bleeding starts.

10

BACK WITH OPTIMISM

So there you are. The complete picture on the concept of joint management as another way to take care of backs that hurt. I trust I have imbued you with a realistic degree of hope.

Of course there will always be backs that are beyond the type of help that we manual therapists can provide, but I am more concerned with those at the other end of the scale who have a totally manageable spinal problem but are completely unaware that such simple, effective help is at hand. Give it a go.

One last thing. It is true that manual mobilisation of joints, not just of spinal joints, is carried out by a relatively small number of therapists throughout the world. Being few in number they are also hard to find. However, every central institute of physiotherapy in whichever country you are will have a register of manual therapists who will have training in this area of specialisation. (Having said that, my name does not appear on one of these lists and probably never will, but it is a good place to start.) Your doctor should know, but, failing that, you should get hold of your telephone directory, look up 'physiotherapists', ring around various practices and ask! Beware of evasive answers. We're good at that, too.

BACKBLOCKS

The BackBlock used in this book can be ordered direct by sending a cheque or money order for £25 (inclusive of postage and packing) to:

Sunsar Blocks
Blenheim Estate Office
Woodstock
Oxon 0XA 1PS
UK

All blocks come with comprehensive instructions on how they should be used.